HEALTH,

HEALING,

WEIGHT LOSS

AND BEAUTY

GUIDE

TABLE OF CONTENT

1. WEIGHT LOSS MYTHS AND FACTS

There are lots of *myths* attached to food and nutrition and its relation to weight reduction which need to be cleared in order to spread awareness and provide step by step guidelines for right choices.

• One such myth is **carbohydrates are culprits behind all weight gain.** Carbohydrates are one of the basic nutrients needed for optimal health and well-being. Foods containing carbohydrates are also good sources of essential vitamins and minerals. Its energy is considered to be readily available whenever needed and can be temporarily stored in the form of glycogen.

• **High protein diets are good for weight reduction**. Moderate protein diets are more safe, useful and cost effective as compared to high protein diets. High protein diets overload the function of kidneys to excrete the waste produced by diets high in protein.

- **Fat free diet can only work.** The diet need to be low in fat. Essential fatty acids are needed in the diet as our body is incapable of producing these inside our body.

- **Drinking too much water can help.** Although water is one of the basic six nutrients needed by our body, but if taken in excess can cause water toxicity.

- **Extremist diet regiments will only help.** A balanced diet needs to be taken at balanced intervals and in balanced amount. Trying to follow extreme paths will not help and can start showing signs of effects of adverse health.

- **Eating before bedtime is not good.** There is no truth in this. The food eaten before bedtime will help in maintaining all the functions and will be a constant source of nourishment during the fast.

- **Unbalanced diet is always needed for weight reduction.** Need to take a well-balanced diet that is low in calories. A diet limiting in calories but not in nutrient is the best policy.

- *Latest weight reduction diets are always better.* Latest weight reduction diets need more fact findings through research. Combination of common sense, wisdom and knowledge should play a more vital role.

- *Staying hungry can help.* Starvation can be harmful and even life threatening. Selecting right food is better than keeping oneself hungry.

- *Pills are replacement for food.* Pills can never be replacement for the abundance of blessings showered upon humanity in the form of all the foods we have. Each food is dependent on the other for all the goodness that it carries.

- *Skinny means healthy.* Being healthy means you should have ideal weight for your height.

- *Dairy and dairy produces make you fat.* Low fat and fat free dairy and dairy products have been found to be helpful in reducing weight.

- ***You need to sacrifice your favorite foods.*** You can reduce weight while sticking with most of your favorite foods.

- ***You need to limit the amount of food.*** You need to limit the calories not the amount. There are few choices while practicing weight reduction. There are a variety of low calorie food items that can be replaced by high calorie food items for your happiness and satisfaction.

- ***Only diet can help me reduce weight.*** A low calorie diet followed by increased activity brings more beneficial results.

- ***You need to go through painful scenario to achieve weight reduction.*** You can enjoy your culinary delights and be contented by making few changes to achieve good results.

- ***Balanced diet cannot be consumed while following weight reduction diet.*** Choosing food from all the basic food groups can help in achieving your goals of eating balanced diets during weight reduction.

• ***Vegetarian diets are better than meat diets.*** Meat is a source of good quality protein, essential vitamins and minerals. To avoid food , nutrient deficiencies to occur during following a weight reducing diet, all food groups need to be given due consideration.

• ***Drinking more water during meals can help in reducing weight.*** Drinking more water during meals can dilute the gastric juices so much that their beneficial effects can be reduced. Drinking enough to satisfy your thirst should be your goal.

• ***Omitting a food group can be beneficial.*** All food groups are important and no food group can be omitted completely. Omitting food groups can only increase the risk factors and can lead to deficiencies.

• ***Artificial sweeteners are good alternative to natural sweeteners.*** Nature cannot be challenged by artificiality. Artificial sweeteners can have negative effects on your body and cannot be an alternative for something natural.

- ***All advertised natural and herbal remedies are safe and reliable.*** Blindly following advertised remedies can be disastrous for your health. Many claims need to be verified by means of research and in-depth study.

- ***Skipping meals can help you reduce weight.*** When you skip a meal you are more likely to eat more in the next meal.

- ***Emphasizing on a single food or a particular pattern rather than on over all approach.*** Varieties of foods are needed to furnish all the nutrients needed by the body.

- ***Drastic reduction of caloric intake can only help.*** Calorie intake should be less than calorie output. Stability is more important than drastic changes.

- ***Each food should be eaten separately.*** Foods consumed in a well-balanced variety can prove to be more beneficial than each eaten separately. Many nutrients are interdependent during digestion and metabolism.

- ***There are magical ways for weight reduction.*** There are no magical ways working for weight reduction without causing any kind of damage to your body. Slow, steady and right approach is the key to success.

- ***White meat is better than red meat.*** Trimmed portion of red meat may provide equal amount of calories as white meat. Red meat also contains more of heme iron needed by many who are anemic.

- ***Nuts are bad because they contain fat.*** Nuts are a source of mono unsaturated and polyunsaturated fatty acids which are considered to be good type fatty acids. Besides, they are also good source of nourishment and fiber and are free from additives and processing.

- ***All fats are bad.*** There are good types of fats e. g., omega 3 fatty acid, omega 6 fatty acid, etc., Essential fatty acids cannot be produced by the body and need to be furnished by a diet.

- ***Everything depends on how much you eat than what you eat.*** More depends on what you are eating than how much you are eating. You can consume five cucumbers and still limit your calorie intake, but if you eat five potatoes than you are in trouble.

• **Listening to everyone's suggestion and following them can help.** Listen to everyone but take your own course of decision and action. One can easily get misguided and distracted trying to follow all the remedies.

• **Certain foods have magical powers to burn your body fat quickly.** There are no such magical foods that will burn your body fat quickly.

• **Following any or all diet pattern can be 100% safe.** Diets which do not possess strong research based foundation cannot be trusted for their safety.

• **You can eat everything if you have increased your activity factor.** Only increasing your physical activity without giving due consideration to your diet will not benefit.

- **No snacking between meals.** You can have snacks between your meals as long as total calorie intake does not exceed your calorie limit.

2. A KETO OR KETOGENIC DIET

A keto diet or a ketogenic diet is a diet which emphasizes on utilization and break down of fats for the energy sources of the body to help achieve weight loss and to provide diet therapy in many diseases, but most commonly to suppress seizures. A typical ketogenic diet is high in total fat, moderate in protein and low in carbohydrates. Among the three energy giving nutrients, it stresses on utilizing fats as a basic source of energy. This diet encourages the process of ketosis through increased fat metabolism. A regular diet is high in carbohydrates, moderate in protein and low in fat.

In a ketogenic diet, 60-80 % of the total calories needed for energy come through fats. This diet has been gaining popularity for weight reduction recently. Initially in the 1920s it was mainly used to provide diet therapy to young patients of epilepsy. Many children who were suffering from seizures had reported to respond positively to this kind of diet and fasting and had reported less incidences of seizure attacks as compared to the ones not taking this diet. Constipation and unpalatable nature of the diet for these kids were the main problems reported. Medium Chain Triglycerides found in abundance in coconut oil was specifically noted for its beneficial properties for such patients.

Its unique metabolic properties has been claimed to be adopted to treat many diseases as well as to reduce weight in a non-traditional way. A ketogenic diet also known as a keto diet is not a well-balanced diet, therefore dietary supplementation and fiber is needed to be taken along with this diet to make it more balanced. Many people who have tried to achieve health benefits through this kind of diet have found its unique properties and have gained set goals.

There have been many positive sides as it helps in catabolizing and breaking down fat deposits in the body. Many benefits have been reported for weight reduction, seizure controlling, improving glycemic index and many more. Still many aspects of this diet need in-depth study and research to fully understand the limitations and boundaries and to fully understand its benefits in many chronic diseases.

To avoid food nutrient deficiencies to occur, nutritional supplements and fiber needed to be added if one is planning to adhere to this kind of diet for a long period of time. In this diet calories from protein and carbohydrates are replaced by calories from fat. Each gram of protein and carbohydrates provide four calories while each gram of fats provides nine calories because fats and foods containing fats are dense in calories, therefore more satiety is achieved by eating less. This diet is dense in calories but deficient in most nutrients, consequently supplementation is needed. The lacking nutrients are necessary to be taken in the form of supplements to avoid deficiency diseases to surface.

During digestive process, carbohydrates enter in the blood stream in the form of glucose. All the extra amount of glucose not wanted for immediate energy need is stored in the form of glycogen in the liver and muscle tissues by the help of a hormone released by the pancreas called insulin. Whenever the blood glucose level rises insulin is released from the pancreas which helps in glycogen synthesis and storage in the liver, muscle tissues and very small amount in the brain and white blood cells. This process is again reversible whenever the need of glucose arises and blood glucose level goes down.

Whenever the blood glucose level goes down the normal range and is not replaced by the diet, this stored glycogen is readily available and converts into glucose and enters in the blood stream maintaining the normal level through a hormone also released by the pancreas called glucagon. Glucagon plays an opposite role of insulin and breaks down the stored glycogen and converts it again to glucose to maintain blood glucose level. The natural system goes on automatically as long as the natural cravings for each food needs are met.

Our brain prefers to use glucose as a form of energy in the presence of glucose. During fasting when all glucose stores are empty or in ketosis, our brain learns to adapt the prevailing conditions and starts utilizing the alternative energy available through fats or break down of fats. Whenever the glycogen storage in the liver gets depleted either by insufficient dietary intake of glucose or inadequate synthesis of glycogen due to lack or absence of insulin, the process of ketogenesis or synthesis of ketone bodies take place. The presence of these ketone bodies causes ketosis which can also be a result of fasting, starvation as well as direct consequences of taking a ketogenic diet.

Ketogenic diet promotes breakdown and utilization of fats for energy and discourages utilization of carbohydrates as a source of energy. Protein in this diet is just enough to maintain growth and repair required in the body. Due to the absence of glycogen stores as a result of low carbohydrates diet, the liver starts to metabolize fats instead to furnish energy. This is promoted by ketogenic diet but can happen naturally during long starvation, stress and fasting conditions. Exercise also supports and helps in this.

Through a ketogenic diet, four parts of total energy requirement comes through fats and only one part is divided between both proteins and carbohydrates. Recipes needed to be developed to make things easier for patients and people who wish to try this diet regimen. What food items can be used liberally, what are moderately restricted and what are strictly restricted. A detailed list of these needed to be provided to them so that they can create their own recipes. Recipe development is an art that does not require much effort. Each individual is different from the other and each one has different activity factor. Each diet needed to be individualized accordingly taking into consideration height, weight, activity factor, likes, dislikes, tolerances, intolerances, preferences, allergies, etc.

Health professionals have been found to be concerned about the proper guidance that needed to be provided to these people. How to start on this diet and what can one expect out of it? How to control and deal with ketosis and how to check serum and urine ketone level? Increasing activity and dealing with the symptoms and whatever needed for proper management. A proper guideline is needed to mentally prepare them of the expectations, tips, benefits and maintenance needed. What needed to be eaten and what needed to be avoided. How to create more palatable recipes? How to sweeten your meal without regular sugar? How to keep oneself motivated and strong? How to have patience and will power? When to exercise and how much is enough?

Many benefits that have been reported are facts that cannot be ignored. Most important benefit that it helps in the breakdown of built in fats and helps in catabolizing adipose tissues cannot be ignored. Adipose tissues are stubborn and are hard to break down. Exercise and increased physical activity do help in breaking down built in fat deposits. Eating a well-balanced diet but with long time intervals also helps in catabolizing fat deposits and can create a situation close to ketosis. Ketogenic diet helps in mobilizing fats to burn up for energy and brain adapts to utilize the energy of fat substrates i.e. ketone bodies. Excess of ketone bodies can get excreted through urine, sweating, breathing and increased physical activity.

Ketosis does also play a protein sparing role. In the presence of ketones, body will not breakdown muscle tissues for the supply of glucose as a source of energy, instead it will utilize the energy from ketones. Body will prefer ketones over glucose and therefore protein would not be oxidized to produce glucose. In normal conditions, whenever blood glucose level goes down and glucose and glycogen supplies are not available, proteins are metabolized to maintain blood glucose level within normal ranges.

In the absence of carbohydrates there are more breakdowns of fats and the body gets adapted to utilizing fats and fat stores in the body instead of relying solely on glucose. As the amount of carbohydrates is lessened in the diet and the stores of glucose and glycogen gets depleted, the insulin level automatically goes down. This causes lipolysis or breakdown of fat and fatty acids leading to ketosis. Our brain in normal conditions consumes around 20% of our total energy output. It prefers to utilize glucose over any other source of energy.

In the absence of carbohydrates, body starts to breakdown muscle tissues to furnish energy needed immediately. Amino acids of protein can be catabolized to provide glucose whenever needed in the absence of carbohydrates. To prevent the process of catabolism and breakdown of muscle tissues during weight reduction and to encourage anabolism or synthesis of muscle tissues and to encourage catabolism or breakdown of adipose tissues or fatty tissues, a diet promoting ketosis is suggested. Ketosis allows the body to get adapted to utilize fats instead of proteins and carbohydrates. Careful planning is needed to bring out the best results needed.

In order to divert body's attention towards utilization of fat stores in the body and to spare proteins for muscle synthesis, a high fat, low carbohydrate and moderate protein diet is suggested. Ketogenic diet needs to be followed after taking into consideration the medical condition of any given individual. It is comparatively a new phenomenon and trend towards weight reduction as historically it has been associated with and used practically to overcome symptoms of epilepsy. More and more claims started to appear for its benefits for many problematic conditions and diseases. It has been found to be beneficial for killing cancer cells, improving glycemic index, found beneficial in type 2 diabetes, controlling seizures, and so on.

More solid studies are needed in this regards to benefit the general public from many therapeutic effects. Awareness programs for understanding the true nature of the diet are needed. Periodic health checks are needed when using this diet practically. Professional supervision and its importance also cannot be ignored. To avoid any kind of danger that might be associated with this, one needs to understand the matter in depth and proper utilization of professional help and guidance whenever and where ever needed. Preparing one-self mentally and knowing why this is suggested, how to go along with it, what the pre-requisites are, what are the limitations and benefits and how it actually works. Deep understanding of the nature of the whole program is looked-for. What one can expect out of it, what tips are desirable, where to look for motivation and help and so on.

Many people due to being handicapped or due to immobile can go for this option. Conditions in which increasing the physical activity or exercise are not advisable or practical, the option of ketogenic diet can work wonders. It should be the last resort not the first one and should never be adopted just for trial and error efforts because switching over diets can be risky. Professional guidance is of real concern here. Preparing oneself emotionally would benefit and help in passing through this phase successfully. One should go back and resume normal diet as soon as possible or after successfully passing through this phase and achieving their dietary goals. Normal diet does not mean over loading your diet with carbohydrates especially simple sugars. Abstinence from alcoholic and carbonated drink is advisable for all.

Ketogenic diet and fasting produces same kind of results. During fasting, a balanced diet necessary to be taken at long intervals. In a ketogenic diet, 3-4 small meals of therapeutic diet plan needed to be followed on a daily basis. It has been suggested by relevant studies that weight reduction does happen through ketogenic diet but mostly it reappears after switching to normal routine once the set goal has been achieved. This has been proved wrong if you stick with the right choices and good habits. Following a ketogenic diet, achieving the good results and then going back again on old habits cannot help. Keeping oneself strong towards good changes and adapting them for life long will show better and long lasting results.

Foods allowed and restricted

What foods needed to be eaten and what foods needed to be avoided when following a ketogenic diet requires understanding of the three basic energy giving nutrients known as the macro nutrients. The only energy giving nutrients among the six major nutrients include carbohydrates, proteins and fats which constitute a major bulk of our daily diet. Both proteins and carbohydrates provide same number of calories per gram i. e. four calories. Fats being dense in calories furnish nine calories per gram.

In order to understand what foods are needed to be eaten and what foods are needed to be avoided in a ketogenic diet, good understanding of food sources of fats, carbohydrates and protein is necessary. Following given list helps in determining the food sources of fats, proteins and carbohydrates.

Food Sources Of Fats

Excellent food sources of fats include butter, margarine, oils, ghee, full cream, lard, mayonnaise, etc.

Good sources of fat include full cream milk, full cream yogurt, prawns, lobster, organ meat, bones broth, lamb, beef, mutton, poultry with skin, eggs, full cream cheese, etc. These food sources are also rich in good quality protein and are poor sources of carbohydrates except milk and milk products which contain lactose sugar.

Significant sources of fats containing foods are also rich in carbohydrates. These include dry fruits, nuts, seeds, avocado, etc.

Food Sources of Protein

Excellent food sources of protein include egg, mutton, beef, fish, lamb, prawns, lobster, poultry, cheese, yogurt, milk, etc.

Good food sources of protein include pulses, beans, tofu, chickpeas, gram, nuts, seeds, gelatin, etc.

Significant sources of protein include corn, rice, wheat, barley, etc.

Poor sources of protein include cucumber, all leafy green vegetables, citrus fruits, yellow squash, radish, mushrooms, onion, turnips, avocado, green pepper, Brussels sprouts, beet root, eggplant, lemon, okra, capsicum, zucchini, garlic, pumpkin, cabbage, tomatoes cauliflower, carrots, asparagus, bean sprouts, broccoli, etc.

Food Sources of Carbohydrate

Excellent food sources of carbohydrates include common sugar, fructose or fruit sugar, honey, brown sugar, molasses, hard candies, etc.

Good food sources of carbohydrates include starchy vegetables and fruits, bananas, potatoes, sweet potatoes, peas, beans, gram, chickpeas, rice, wheat, barley, sorghum, millet, corn, mango, cheeko, etc.

Fair sources of carbohydrates include milk and milk products, green leafy vegetables, non-starchy vegetables, butter squash, avocado, tomatoes, cucumber, ice berg, cabbage, green pepper, zucchini, Brussels sprouts, eggplant, lemon, pumpkin, asparagus, carrots, cauliflower, capsicum, onion, bean sprouts, turnips, mushroom, garlic, radish, beet root, okra, etc.

List of Food items that can be used to create recipes for a ketogenic diet include the following.

To create recipes for a ketogenic diet, it require techniques of mixing foods with each other with limited choices in such a way that their palatability is increased and individual needs are met. This needs pure challenging situation and very good planning. A ketogenic diet promotes the excess usage of fats and fat rich sources of foods therefore these diets must be rich in butter, cream, ghee, margarine, olive oil, coconut cream, peanut butter, canola oil, palm oil, sesame oil, macadamia, coconut butter, flax seed oil, lard, avocado oil, creamy salad dressings, mayonnaise, butter cream frosting, cream cheese, coconut oil, etc. Fat selection should be according to individual tolerance and intolerance, likes and dislike and preferences. Any fat which is found to be intolerable must be replaced by other fats and oils. Olive oil, coconut oil, coconut cream and avocado oil is advisable for their therapeutic properties.

As ketogenic diet is low in carbohydrates, and therefore low carbohydrate vegetables can be used in good combination and different seasonings and methods of cooking can be applied to create and develop mouth-watering dishes and recipes. Vegetables that can be used include avocado, spinach, lettuce, fresh cilantro, fresh mint, parsley, cabbage, fresh basil, ice berg, summer squash, Brussels sprouts, cauliflower, green pepper, zucchini, black olives, mushrooms, and fair amount of carbohydrates from the list of fair sources of carbohydrates can be used.

A ketogenic diet is moderate in protein so moderate amount of excellent sources of protein must be included. Good sources and significant sources of protein needed to be avoided as they are good sources of carbohydrates as well and basic idea behind a ketogenic diet is to have a diet that is low in carbohydrates to promote ketosis and break down and utilization of fats in the body. Beef, poultry, fish, prawns, lobster, organ meat, mutton, cheese, yogurt, egg, lamb, etc. can be used in moderation and in combination with different low carbohydrate vegetables to increase and improve palatability of the diet. Each individual likes and dislikes needed to be given due consideration as well as food tolerances and intolerances. Fattier cuts of meat and chicken with skin needed to be used where ever possible.

Different ways of cooking e. g. baking, stewing, barbecuing, frying, steaming, can be used to make food more likable and palatable. Different combinations of color to improve garnishing can make food more appealing and improves its acceptability. Different herbs and spices can be used to improve the flavor of foods e. g. basil, parsley, ginger powder, garlic powder, black pepper, cinnamon powder, etc. Use of various available sauces and flavor enhancers to develop creative recipes can be pure fun e. g. tomato ketchup, soy sauce, Worcestershire sauce, mustard sauce, barbeque sauce, etc.

As ketogenic diet being low in carbohydrates it does not allow the usage of corn or other flours to be used as thickening agents. Instead we can use the alternatives available. Coconut flour, cream cheese, whipped cream, heavy-cream, gelatin-powder, macadamia nuts-flour, almond flour, pecans flour, coconut cream, peanut butter, coconut butter, etc. can all help in making gravies, soups and sauces that could be used in good combinations for better results.

In a ketogenic diet energy should mostly come through 60-80 % fats, 15-25% protein and 5-15 % carbohydrates. Total carbohydrate intake should be less than 60 grams. Protein intake could vary between 1-2 gm. for each kilogram of body weight. Rest of the energy should come through fats. Around 20-25 gm. of fiber should be added daily to make up for a low carbohydrates diet and consequently low fiber diet. Flax seed can be incorporated into various recipes for its high fiber content. Salads with rich dressings can be helpful in furnishing of more fiber and increasing the fat content of salads. Multivitamin supplements needed to be taken regularly.

Reaching ketosis through ketogenic diet

Whenever our liver is short of energy from carbohydrates, it starts metabolizing fats for energy as an alternative source. During the catabolism or break down of fats to furnish energy ketone bodies are produced which causes ketosis. Ketosis always occurs inside our body whenever our body is deficient of energy from carbohydrate sources but can also happen due to some medical problem and because of taking a ketogenic diet. During the process of lipolysis breakdown of fats occur and triglycerides are broken down to provide three molecules of fatty acid chains and one molecule of glycerol.

The fatty acids produced by this process can be utilized by our body as a secondary source of energy in the absence of glucose. Breakdown of fats and fatty acids are promoted by fasting, exercising or increased physical activity, starvation and ketogenic diet. The body physically gets to start adapting to utilizing the fats. Fat stored in our body in the form of adipose tissues, is being metabolized to furnish energy to the body. The breakdown of fatty tissues in our body helps us in saving our muscle tissues. Weight is being lost at the expense of the built in fats and not at the expense of built in muscles. Increased physical activity, fasting, starvation and ketogenic diet all are beneficial in achieving this to some extent.

The utilizing of fats instead of carbohydrates results in the production of ketone bodies and the state of ketosis. Our liver is responsible for the synthesis of ketone bodies. Ketone bodies are important because our brain which consumes around 20 % of all our energy need prefers glucose over any other available energy source. But in the absence of glucose it is unable to utilize long chain fatty acids as they are bound with albumin protein and are unable to furnish energy to the brain. These ketone bodies produced can be utilized by the brain for energy.

Our brain consumes high amount of energy as compared to the amount of mass it possess and we cannot even blame it as it never sleeps. Even when we are fast asleep, our brain keeps functioning and helps us to digest the food that we have eaten, circulate all the blood around our body and keep all internal functions to work automatically without our involvement and any effort. So the brain does deserve lots of energy that it needs.

Ketone bodies are acidic in nature and therefore excess of these in our blood can be harmful for people who are suffering from diabetes and needs treatment to overcome ketoacidosis which could lead to diabetic coma and even death. A normal healthy body is capable of handling this and maintaining the blood pH level within normal ranges. Ketoacidosis can happen mostly in type I diabetes but can also happen in type II diabetes cases rarely. Excess of ketones in the blood and urine for a long period of time can damage internal organ e. g. kidneys and liver. Therefore extra water needed to be taken in order to flush out these through urine, breath and sweating and to free the body of its toxicity. Water also helps in diluting these.

Signs of ketosis and its testing

Excess ketone bodies produced during stress, starvation, fasting or a ketogenic diet can start accumulating in the blood stream causing typical fruity odor in breath and passing out extra ketones in the urine. A urine sample can be tested to find out and evaluate the presence of ketone bodies in urine at home level using specific strips needed.

Following are some of the reported signs and symptoms associated with ketosis.

- Presence of ketone bodies in urine.

- Fruity odor in breath.

- Extra thirst.

- Head ache, fatigue and tiredness.

- Frequent urination.

- High energy level and clear thinking.

- Weakness and dizziness.

- Stomach ache, nausea, and sleep problems.

- Unusual taste in mouth.

- Cold feet and hand.

Ketosis is not a harmful condition for a healthy human being and through ketogenic diet it is used to maximize the breakdown of stored fat in the body. Initial stage of reaching ketosis can be disturbing and may be a cause for discomfort but the signs and symptoms start to subside as the body gets adapted to the new energy sources. Urine sample may not always show the presence of ketone bodies and can be misleading. Excess intake of water or utilization of ketones during increased physical activity can be the causes for misleading urine sample. Drinking extra water may dilute the urine to give wrong report.

A person going through ketosis may find it to be an unpleasant experience due to the body's reaction and also due to the unpalatable nature of the diet. Very high levels of ketones needed to be avoided as they can have damaging effects on the liver and kidneys and therefore can be toxic. Extra ketones can be removed by drinking extra water, breathing it out through lungs and using it up by increasing the physical activity.

Ketogenic diet for diabetics

Diabetes is a chronic disease in which the metabolism of carbohydrates is affected due to inefficiency or total failure of pancreas to produce insulin or resistance of body cells to insulin. There are three types of diabetes.

In type I diabetes also known as juvenile or insulin dependent diabetes, insulin is needed to be injected with intervals as pancreas are totally unable to produce this. This type of diabetes is controlled through insulin injections, diet and exercise.

In type II diabetes the body is able to produce insulin but the cells of the body are resistant to it. Therefore patients are treated through hypoglycemic drugs, diet and exercise. These patients may at times need doses of insulin to control blood sugar. Type III diabetes occur during pregnancy and could be controlled by diet and exercise. Around one in five may need to take hypoglycemic agents.

A ketogenic diet can be allowed to be followed by patients suffering from diabetes under controlled conditions and proper guidance and supervision of professionals concerned. Ketoacidosis is a serious condition in which a diabetic patient can develop signs and symptoms of diabetic coma which could be life threatening if proper medical care is not provided in a timely manner.

A normal healthy body is capable of maintaining the pH of the blood. People who are suffering from diabetes are incapable of reversing ketoacidosis and need external medical intervention. Over nutrition is also one of the causes of diabetes and eating in limitation is very important to avoid obesity leading to many chronic diseases.

Diabetic ketoacidosis and its symptoms sometime may appear within a day. Signs and symptoms may include loss of appetite, abdominal pain, confusion, weakness, shortness of breath, nausea, fatigue, vomiting, dry skin, excessive thirst, dry mouth, low blood pressure, fruity smell in breath, difficulty in breathing, excessive urination, etc. Testing the blood for sugar level and urine for ketone level can confirm the signs and let the person suffering know when to consult a physician. At times emergency care may be needed to avoid coma or even death. These patients might require insulin, rehydration and electrolyte intake.

Health benefits and expectations

Before starting a ketogonic diet one need to get aware of what to expect while passing through this phase practically for its benefits. How it could benefit and preparing mentally to handle the initial time period specially those who feel carbohydrates are inseparable part of their lives is very important. A ketogenic diet is all about changing a way of how you eat your diet. Initial time period can be rough till the body gets adapted to the new diet regimen.

Its beneficial effects for patients suffering from epilepsy are well known. This diet has been found to be lessening the attacks of seizures and in many cases eliminating seizures.

Keeping the blood glucose levels low and ketones level high have been found to be beneficial for cancer patients as it has been reported to kill cancer cells.

Many people suffering from type II diabetes have experienced better control over blood glucose level and feel there are many benefits attached to it.

Decreased level of joint pain, controlled blood pressure, and lessening of heart burn are few other reported benefits.

Weight loss through reduction in adipose tissues instead of muscle tissues is one more known advantage.

Other known benefits which still need more studies and evidence include Alzheimer's, Parkinson's, narcolepsy, brain trauma, amyotrophic lateral sclerosis, acne, brain cancer, polycystic ovarian syndrome, etc.

The transition time period from normal diet to ketogenic diet lasts for few days when the body gets adapted to a new primary source of energy i. e. fats can cause few disturbing symptoms. These symptoms may include headache, irritability, fatigue, weakness and most of these symptoms may subside within a week or so. The serum, urine and breath ketone level will increase. Long term usage may affect your serum lipid profile which could even be positive. Serum lipid profile and blood glucose level needed to be checked at least once a month to keep them within normal ranges.

In the beginning within two weeks of ketogenic diet, dramatic weight loss may occur due to depleted stores of glycogen from liver and muscle tissues consequently loss of water held by these cells. Total water loss will be proportional to the total muscle mass. Ketogenic diet has been gaining popularity since last twenty years for weight loss and its therapeutic properties for many chronic diseases.

While following a ketogenic diet, serum ketone level must not cross the borderline and therefore needs regular checking. Increased blood acidity could have damaging effect on the liver and kidneys.

A ketogenic diet has been found to be especially beneficial for brain functions and treatment of brain diseases. It has historically been proven to eliminate or decrease seizures. Our brain contains high amount of fats as compared to other organs and therefore consume high energy as well.

Adaptation to this diet may take from one week to twelve weeks. A person may pass through the phase of fat phobia once adjusted fully to this diet.

Success tips

Increasing physical activity

Increasing physical activity in addition to following a diet regimen will help in losing weight even faster and helping in developing muscle tissues. Half an hour of brisk walking, cycling, swimming or jogging all are beneficial.

Increasing intake of fluids

Increasing water and fluid intake can help in excreting extra load of ketone bodies and relieving the body of toxic waste especially in hot weather conditions when there is increased physical activity and consequently increased sweating.

Decreasing intake of alcohol

Alcoholic drinks also contribute to energy so must be discontinued and they can also cause carbohydrate overload.

Be more creative with recipes, keep your spirits high, avoid caffeinated drinks, keep yourself motivated, keep a check on urine and blood ketone level which needed to be maintained, keep a track of weight loss, understand and adhere to the diet protocol, etc.

If sticking to a regular or standard ketogenic diet is difficult, one can try a cyclical ketogenic diet. In this one need to follow a ketogenic diet from Monday to Friday and on weekends it is allowed to take a carbohydrates overload. In this exercise is needed on weekdays only and can rest on weekends and have carbohydrates overload and stores for the whole week on weekends. If cyclical ketogenic diet is not suitable then one can go for targeted ketogenic diet. In targeted ketogenic diet 25-50 gm. of carbohydrate is allowed before a work out.

Good understanding of what is needed to be eaten and what needed to be avoided is very important. Keeping vigilant to various signs and symptoms of any kind of health problem or concern should not be ignored.

Losing and maintaining weight

Losing and maintaining weight on a ketogenic diet is very important and one need to keep oneself motivated towards it for life long results. How many calories a person will need on a keto diet will depend primarily on individual height, weight and activity factor and on the fact of calorie input and calorie output. One pound of weight is lost when we take 3500 calories less in the diet than we utilize it e.g. if some ones calorie intake is 1200 and calorie output is 1700 then this person will lose one lb. per week if he sticks on taking 500 calories less for one whole week. In order to increase your intake you have to first start catabolizing more which can be achieved by increasing physical activity.

Regular brisk walk, swimming, cycling or any form of aerobic exercise need to be part of daily routine. Your daily energy expenditure will depend on your metabolic rate. Your metabolic rate is high when you are active and it slows down when you are sedentary. Lessening the use of machinery in our daily lives to accomplish various tasks, and making better use of our own efforts which could be easily achieved through little exertion all can have beneficial response towards increased physical activity at our own home level. In this way you do not have to spend extra time, effort or money to leave your home and visit a gym. Light to moderate activity could be achieved through this way which is required initially. Later on when your body gets fully adapted to the new diet then you can plan for more active and vigorous exercises and may schedule your gym visits on regular basis close to your neighborhood.

How much body fat you must lose will depend on the percentage of existing fat in your body of your total body weight. Increasing physical activity in addition to following a strict ketogenic diet regimen will give more beneficial and long lasting results. Losing faith, spirit and motivation during initial difficult time period will only leave you in the middle of nowhere.

Correct understanding of suitable ratio of macro nutrients needed is essential. Good understanding of good, fair and poor sources of macronutrients is required. 50 gm. of carbohydrates can easily be consumed in a minute in the form of a candy. The same amount of carbohydrates can be distributed in the whole day in the form of high fiber non starchy vegetables. Protein intake can also vary according to individual height and weight and activity factor. During increased physical activity or vigorous exercising you may be able to consume a more liberal intake of good quality protein as these will be utilized for muscle anabolism.

One can start from 50 % of calories from fats. Watch for one week and let the body get adapted to high fat content. Choose only those fats which you feel your body tolerates well. Fats can be consumed easily if incorporated in soups or emulsions. Emulsions can be prepared using nut flours. Drinking lots of broth prepared from bones will help in reducing dehydration and any deficiency of sodium. Addition of little lemon juice will help in preventing potassium deficiency.

Rest and sleep is of utmost importance during following a ketogenic diet. It helps in keeping the body in good working condition especially when we have started a new diet altogether. Pay more attention to your body and needs of your body. Respond to its need whenever needed. If you feel thirsty do not ignore. Ketones can cause toxicity and can have damaging effect if you do not drink enough water or fluids needed. These toxins like others needed to be relieved through urine so you stay healthy. So drink water whenever you feel thirsty.

First week on a ketogenic diet may be difficult so be prepared for it from the beginning. This is temporary because your body is passing through an adaptation phase. You have introduced a fat diet to it and it is trying to adjust to it. One very important thing to remember is not to cheat. Please do not cheat yourself. It will not help you in any way as the whole system will get disrupted. During ketogenic diet the blood sugar level need to remain at lower levels and carbohydrates are not the only culprits to raise sugar level. Proteins are made up of amino acids and these can convert to glucose to maintain blood sugar level. Fats can also contribute to this. Glycerol a metabolite of fats can turn into glucose.

This diet has been found to be helpful for mental alertness and improved mental capabilities. Patiens play an important part in this diet because weight loss can be slow and steady. Rapid weight loss is never good and therefore should not be our goal. Weight loss may vary from person to person depending upon their genetic makeup, body metabolic rate, physical-activity, sleeping pattern and food ingestion. Each individual is unique in his makeup and individual response to this diet will also be unique.

From the beginning till around three weeks into this diet people may find it difficult to exercise. For these three weeks light exercise is recommended. Later on the intensity of exercise may be increased. Keeping your insulin level low will help you in breaking down built in fat and will discourage anabolism of fatty tissues. Keep checking your weight on weekly or fortnightly basis. Make a target goal where you want to reach. Calculate your ideal body weight for your height. For 5 feet, 100 lbs. for females and 106lbs. for males are ideal. With one inch increase in height we have to add 5lbs. for females and 6lbs. for males. For each inch of extra height, keep on adding the pounds. Ten percent above or below the ideal will also come within the ideal. Any variance more than this or less than this will be considered overweight or underweight. If someone is more than 20 % of his ideal body weight he will come under obese category.

Do not eat when you are not hungry but only when you feel hungry. Be patient and avoid artificial sweeteners as much as possible. Sleep more and do not take unnecessary stress. Proceed wisely with your diet therapy. Avoid alcoholic drinks and fruits. Instead take fibers, minerals and vitamin supplement. Increase physical activity smartly. High fat content of ketogenic diet will help in suppressing your hunger you need not force feed yourself. There is lot of built in energy inside your body which need to be burnt. Let that energy take care of the energy needed by the body.

According to one authentic study people burn more energy on low carbohydrate diet while resting. Rest and sleep helps the body to get adjusted to things easily.

Measure your waist circumference on weekly basis. It is also advisable to keep a track of your blood pressure and serum lipid profile once a month or once in two months.

You may lose 1-6 pounds during the first week and 1 pound on weekly basis after the first week. But this may vary with individual cases.

Maintaining your weight will require you to change your eating habits and lifestyle. Following most of the rules of healthy living, eating and adapting may have far reaching implications that may prove to improve overall health.

There are three types of ketogenic diet standard ketogenic diet, cyclic ketogenic diet and targeted kitogenic diet. A standard ketogenic diet does not allow any overload of carbohydrates. A person can be active as much as possible but it has been a known fact that people keep losing weight on this diet even if they do not feel they have enough stamina for exercising and if they do not exercise. In cyclical ketogenic diet a person can do work out twice or thrice a week during the week days and is allowed a load of carbohydrates during the weekend. During weekend a person can take rest and no need for any exercise. In targeted ketogenic diet a person can work out during the week and before working out he is given 25-50 gm. of carbohydrates load for stamina.

This diet is famous among people who are either unable to exercise or people who do not like to work out. It is a known fact that this diet work wonders even without exercising and the results are more long lasting as it deals with the base line of dealing with the problem of wrong kind of fat deposits inside the body. It helps in reducing these built in hulks and attacks them with a purpose. It has been looked all around by professionals for its safety and till now has been declared to be safe enough to be practiced. Keeping a check on ketone levels, drinking enough water, resting and sleeping well, increasing activity whenever easily possible and sticking with the diet regimen will help and bear fruitful results. Keeping your patience intent and not letting it go and keeping self-motivated will help.

Do not keep a check on your weight on daily basis and do not measure your waistline every now and then. Ketogenic diet is not magic and will take its time to bring good and fruitful results. Get support from people around and talk out your problem and discuss with people who have tried this diet. Pay more attention on your interests and less on thinking about food and do not think about foods you are not allowed to eat. Once you get tempted and eat out of your diet pattern you may come out of ketosis and it will take few days for you to get back again to ketosis. Whenever you are tempted to eat something sweet and feel you are having a sweet tooth then select foods which are prepared by using artificial sweeteners e. g. diet jelly, etc. just to curb the temptation.

Frequently asked questions

Q.   Are all low carbohydrate diets ketogenic diets?

A.   No, not all low carbohydrate diets are ketogenic diets.

Q. What is a ketogenic diet?

A. A ketogenic diet promotes the utilization of fat energy over protein or carbohydrate energy.

Q. How does it work to benefit?

A.   It emphasizes on the catabolism or break-down of adipose-tissues rather than muscle-tissues.

Q. Is it safe to use?

A. It has been tried and tested and for a healthy individual it does not pose any health risks.

Q.   Do we have to take it through-out our life time?

A.   You need to stick to it till your ideal weight to height or set-goals have been achieved.

Q. Is it safe in all conditions?

A.   No, it is not safe in all conditions. It is not advisable to pursue this diet in chronic liver or kidney disease. Also, it is not safe during pregnancy and lactation.

Q. Can I reduce weight through this diet?

A. Yes, this diet is suitable for weight reduction.

Q.   How do we distinguish this diet from other diets?

A. This diet is high in fats, adequate in proteins and low in carbohydrates.

Q. In how many days do we achieve ketosis?

A. In around two days' time.

Q. Can I increase physical activity along with this diet?

A. Yes, exercise along with ketogenic diet is advisable.

3. HEALTH AND HEALING POWER OF COCONUTS AND COCONUT OIL

Coco is a Spanish word that means monkey face. Resemblance of coconut with its three indentations and hairy nut to monkey's face; it started to be known as coconut. Coconut has innumerable health benefits and uses. Due to coconut's long and much respected history, around 1 / 3 of human population around the world depend to a great extent in one way or the other on its supplies and production. 'The tree of life' was the name given to it by the Pacific Islanders and historically it was considered to have a cure for all diseases. Recent studies on this have revealed many hidden secrets for its healing powers. For thousands of years it has been used to treat many illnesses and diseases besides being used as a component of food.

It has proved not only to cure diseases but helpful in preventing many diseases. Other than these, coconut oil has been proved to be beneficial in different industrial uses due to its high gelling temperature and viscosity. Its long shelf life due to high resistance to rancidity makes it easier to store it for long period of time. To improve shelf life hydrogen molecule is added through a process called hydrogenation. This process increases the saturation of unsaturated fatty acids i. e. mono unsaturated and polyunsaturated fatty acids. Partial hydrogenation of these leads to synthesis of trans-fatty acids. Trans fatty acids are responsible for causing cardiovascular diseases and conditions leading to it.

Therefore, coconut oil in its original natural condition is not at all bad for the heart but artificial and synthetic processing of it leads to making hydrogenated coconut oil saturated enough to have any kind of negative effects on dietary intakes leading to health problems. Virgin coconut oil and extra virgin coconut oil are free from trans-fats. These oils needed to be incorporated in all kinds of meal planning, beauty products, massaging and medicinal properties for their innumerable benefits and powerful natural effects.

It has been noted that people of Sri Lanka who consume high amounts of coconut and coconut products have one of the lowest heart disease rates. Due to this blaming coconut as the cause of heart disease is absolutely wrong and baseless when the main culprit is hydrogenation and saturation processes just to improve the flavors and increase its shelf life and consequently gaining more financial benefits. Scientific name for coconut is cocos nucifera. Coconut is slightly sweet in flavor and a dry kernel contains around 60 %- 65 % fats.

Coconut oil and components of coconut oil have typical distinguishing factors making them altogether highly valued due to these. Coconut oil has been used for centuries for its unique properties in many parts of the world and the wisdom of the wise kept on passing the goodness sealed within from one generation to the next. Due to its true medicinal value, a tree of coconut is considered a symbol of life and is a great source of coconut meat, milk, juice and oil. Coconut juice is a purest of all juices and sealed with perfection to furnish all the goodness inside. Its goodness has not been felt only inside the body but outer application through massage and in beauty products have been proved.

In medicine its component in the form of medium chain triglycerides commonly known as MCT oil has proven record that no other oil can compete. MCT oil can be added to naso-gastric feeds commonly known as NG feeds. It has many proven uses in industries as well where other types of fats failed to achieve the same results and this is only due to its unique composition which makes it different from the rest. It also possesses one more distinguishing quality among plant sources of fats and oils of having longest shelf life. It lasts longer than other oils and does not get rancid easily.

It has achieved a status of being a source of food and medicine among the people from all around the world speaking different languages, having different cultures, belonging to different religions and adhering to various traditions. Its beneficial uses have been traditionally passed on from one generation to another. 1 tbsp. Of coconut oil furnishes around 117 calories while 1 tbsp. of other oils furnishes around 135 calories. Therefore it is the only known fat that has lower caloric value as compared to either butter or any other hydrogenated vegetable oil source.

Coconut oil contains 92 % saturated fat. Pure virgin coconut oil can be solid, semi-solid or liquid depending upon the room temperature. It is made up of various fatty acids and contains lauric acid, myristic acid and capric acid. It may contain other beneficial chemical sources of plants that may get discovered through studies.

Only recently it has been studied in the light of science and scientific facts. Its real goodness has been rediscovered through scientific investigations and procedures. This ongoing process has been helpful in distinguishing between myths and facts. Scientific understanding knew that there is some truth behind the words of the wise based on centuries. Many researchers due to this dedicated their time, money and efforts to unfold the hidden truth. Many studies have been conducted in the area but still many more are needed to fully understand its potential for being unique in its own sense.

Presence of lauric acid in coconut oil in abundance makes it anti-bacterial, anti-viral, anti-fungal and anti-protozoal. Coconut fat contains around 50 % lauric acid which is a medium chain fatty acid. Monolaurin is being produced from lauric acid inside a human body which acts like anti-bacterial, anti-viral and anti-protozoal. Monoglycerides of lauric acid have shown even better results and are more effective than the fatty acid itself. Good thing about mono-laurine is that it does not destroy the gut bacteria which are desirable but only attacks the pathogenic micro-organisms.

Coconut fat contains about 6-7 % capric acid which is another kind of medium chain fatty acids. Inside a human body it is formed into mono-caprin which has shown to have antiviral effects against HIV. Capric acid has also been found to possess qualities of anti-microbial.

Coconut oil is one of the few natural plant sources of saturated fat and the kind of fat it possess is helpful in reducing the bad type cholesterol and increasing the good type cholesterol naturally. Types of fatty acids found in coconut oil have been recognized to have specific natural health renewal system that needs in-depth study and understanding. Some of the naturally occurring saturates found in coconut oil are found to be more beneficial than some of the unsaturated from other sources.

This leads to a conclusion that how could nature be challenged by labeling foods to be either good or bad. Therefore, all foods are good if eaten in balance and given due consideration to wide variety. Each food contains some kind of goodness missing from the others. Extremism in food intake and liking and disliking leads to deficiencies or over nourishment leading to obesity and consequently to many diseases.

Using coconut and its oil as wholesome or utilizing its various beneficial components e. g. lauric acid, capric acid or MCT , all have proved to be beneficial in one way or the other for many conditions and eliminating or reducing the effects of many diseases. It helps in soothing sore throat, works as a lip balm and provides relief from ear infection.

Virgin coconut oil has been found to provide protection to liver from various effects of drugs. .

It has also been found to be beneficial in either eliminating or reducing problems associated with many chronic diseases and helping in providing alternative natural therapies without any due side effects. Many diseases and conditions in which it has been tried and tested and found to be of great benefits include GERD, chronic sinusitis, heart problems, Alzheimer, hemorrhoid, cancer, diabetes, psoriasis, gall bladder diseases, bladder infection, flu, athletic foot, ring worm, arthritis, Parkinson, etc. Each individual is unique and therefore each one's response to coconut therapy may be different and we also cannot expect coconut to be the cure for all diseases but one thing is certain that it is only a part of a diet and do not carry any type of side effects with it.

Coconut oil has also been found to be helpful in increasing the absorption of minerals and vitamins and other nutrients from the gut e. g. calcium, magnesium, fat soluble vitamins A, D, E, K, beta-carotene and few amino acids. In this way it is indirectly responsible for reducing undernourishment and deficiencies.

Coconut oil can be consumed through dietary intake. Adding it in many dishes can create great recipes. It can also be consumed directly through tea spoon full or table spoon full once or twice daily respectively. Its daily intake is important for good health, protection from infection and to avoid many health problems, conditions and diseases.

It has also been found to prevent stretch marks of pregnancy, support thyroid function and provide relief from psoriasis, eczema, varicose veins, depression, autism, allergy symptoms, cellulites, anxiety, baby rash, sleep disorders, decreased mental alertness, etc.

Coconut oil has high smoking point and it also possesses anti insect repellent properties. It improves memory, regulates hormones, reduces wrinkles, heals wounds, reduces epileptic seizures, dissolves kidney stones, improves digestion, etc.

A coconut palm is from a family of Arecaceae and in the genus cocos it is the only accepted specie.

It is commonly found in the tropical and subtropical areas. Due to its versatility of various uses of its different parts, it is well known for its high value.

Coconut is being consumed in many parts of the world as staple food. Coconut fruit contains large amount of water when mature and are different from other fruits. Immature coconut fruit contains tender nuts and could be consumed as a drink. The hard outside shell can be used as charcoal. The dried coconut flesh is called copra. Oil derived from the hard nut can be used for cooking, frying and baking. Coconut milk and cream can also be used in a variety of ways in cookery.

Coconut oil is also used in a variety of ways in the manufacture of soaps and cosmetics. Coconut water, a clear liquid is a refreshing drink. The leaves, husks, shell and its wood is used to manufacture many goods and products. Countries which are great suppliers of coconut and its products include Philippines, Malaysia, Indonesia, India, Maldives, Polynesia, and southern Asia. It is also commonly found in South America, Pacific Island, Hawaii and Florida.

All parts of a coconut tree is beneficial in one way or the other and therefore its tree is supposed to supply everything needed for a living. Coconut fruit has a variety of food uses e. g. coconut meat, cream, milk, sugar, water and oil. The shell is also utilized as a bowl, dish or cup. The fibers of seeds are used in the making of brushes, mats, fishnets and rope.

It takes around one whole year for a coconut to mature but the tree blooms thirteen times per year. Coconuts are continuously formed and harvest is available the year round. An average harvest from one tree is 60 coconuts and many trees yield three times this amount. It is considered to be a drupe and not a nut. Some coconut trees are tall and some are dwarfs. Fruits from dwarfs are eaten fresh while fruits from tall trees are used for the supply of coconut oil and fiber.

The dwarf trees tend to account for only 5 percent of coconut. They are self-fertilizing, produce rounded sweet fruit, are being self-pollinated and have domesticated traits. It is difficult to track the origins of cultivation due to the long history of human interaction with coconut

Many common coconut oil myths are attached to it due to miss-understandings and many due to artificial hype created by vested interest groups for various economy factors related to it. Whatever the reasons behind one thing is certain that due to this many have been deprived of its so many blessings showered upon humanity by nature's gift and will keep on depriving if kept in darkness. One more reason leading towards this is by artificial saturation process of hydrogenation leading to reduced beneficial effects and increased harmful effects which could easily be avoided. But this has been the most neglected issue not only towards coconut oil but all sorts of vegetable oils. Strict policy development on universal basis and adherence to it is urgently required by the policy makers to avoid further damage occurring due to this.

Hydrogenation process is the culprit behind synthetic saturation of oils leading to production of trans- fatty acids. Trans-fatty acids have proven record of causing all sorts of diseases. No one would like to compromise on health just for the sake of the flavor of the food. There are thousands of ways to improve the flavor without compromising on health. Besides improving the flavor, hydrogenation process is also responsible to increase the viscosity and shelf life. Increased viscosity also leads to increased market acceptability and majority of the public being ignorant finds these more appealing. Many people start blaming the oil instead of the processing behind. For this, more awareness programs are needed in all the nook and corner of the world.

Only to make these oils more marketable and gain more profits these kinds of processes and tactics are applied without giving due consideration to its harmful effects on humanity.

This is happening throughout the world and no particular area can be blamed but each one is affected even after knowing. The process of hydrogenation of oils needed to be banned if we want the chances of decreased obesity, hypertension, cardiovascular and many other diseases to increase. Many food authorities have taken measurable actions against it and many are requiring proper labeling of the content of foods to decrease incidences of these diseases.

There is no credible scientific support available against coconut or coconut oil causing any kind of negative effects. It is untrue to suggest coconut does not possess healing powers when it has been time and again proven record through research studies showing it to have natural antibiotic and anti-oxidative properties. Just black listing it due to its natural saturation properties is not enough to label it heart enemy oil.

One myth involving coconut oil and its consumption is associated with weight gain and it is believed mistakenly that it helps in weight gain and obesity which is not at all true. Medium chain fatty acids present in coconut oil helps in increasing the metabolic rate and energy is being consumed at a higher level and more energy is spent and released and more fat is being utilized.

Coconut oil does not raise the bad type cholesterol and protects the heart towards developing atherosclerosis or developing conditions leading to heart diseases.

Many people also believe that coconut oil irritates skin which is not at all true. It actually protects the skin from all kinds of itching and irritation. It helps in soothing the skin in case of inflammation caused by insect bites, sun burn, allergies, bruises and reaction of drugs. The anti-microbial properties associated with coconut oil helps in healing wounds and fight off infection.

One more myth attached with coconut oil is that it is sweet and cannot be consumed by diabetics. Coconut oil does not contain glucose and is not at all sweet. In fact this oil promotes secretion of insulin from the pancreas and reduces the chances to develop diabetes greatly.

Many people also believe that coconut oil is thick in cold climatic conditions and do not get easily absorbed by the skin. In fact this is totally untrue as it becomes liquid as it comes into contact with the skin temperature and gets readily absorbed by the skin and is preferred for massaging and tanning.

Many myths are also associated with its shelf life. As it is obtained from coconut which is high in moisture content it has short shelf life and gets rancid easily. This is untrue and coconut oil has long shelf life and do not get rancid easily. In fact it has the longest shelf life amongst most of the oils from plant origins. If unopened it may last for three to four years and opened bottle can last for at least two years. If refrigerated and unopened can even last for eight to ten years without getting rancid.

One more myth associated with this oil is that it tastes bad. Most of the people who have tasted it believe that it tastes very good. One can fry a thing in coconut oil and try out and will understand how good it tastes.

Coconut oil has been able to recover from blameworthy situation of being heart enemy to heart friendly. Just because it was naturally saturated it was thought that it might have negative effects on our heart which was proved to be totally wrong after various studies and researches found out the truth. The kind of saturated fat it is and many of its constituents helps in decreasing many kinds of diseases mainly cardiac and obesity.

The presence of lauric acid in coconut oil helps in increasing the serum HDL level which is good type cholesterol. Numerous health benefits of coconut and its oil and derivatives of its oils are well known through population studies especially its role in decreasing heart diseases and increasing resistance to many diseases. It has some inbuilt chemical power that makes it differ from the rest and most probably its unique fatty acid composition makes it hard to ignore for its all beneficial medicinal properties known from centuries. Many studies have proved it to be beneficial in many conditions but many still are under way.

Coconut oil has also been seen to have a cholesterol lowering action by converting it to pregenolone. Pregenalone is a molecule which is a precursor for many hormones that a human body needs. Most of the therapeutic value of coconut lies in its fat content.

Abnormal thyroid function can be a cause for increase in bad type cholesterol. Coconut oil helps in normalizing and regulating the thyroid function. It also helps in reducing stress and sore throat.

Coconut oil has also been associated with having an effect of lowering the amount of belly fat. Abdominal fat stores are associated with cardiovascular problems and this fat is even difficult to lose.

Although 92 % of naturally occurring coconut oil is saturated fat, but it has been found to provide protection against heart attacks and strokes. It has also been associated with giving strength to bones.

Non hydrogenated naturally occurring coconut oil helps in improving the cholesterol profile of blood.

According to various researches based on population studies people who have been traditionally consuming large amounts of coconut and coconut oil have low to very low incidences of cardiovascular diseases and their serum cholesterol level remain within normal ranges.

Studies have also revealed the presence of Medium Chain Fatty Acids MCFA in coconut oil for being responsible for protection against heart diseases.

Many studies have also revealed that coconut consumption has been resulting in lowering heart diseases, improving cholesterol levels, lowering fat deposits, increasing rate of survival, reducing blood clot tendency, lessening uncontrolled free radicals in cell, improving anti-oxidant reserves, decreasing incidences of cardiovascular diseases, etc.

Atherosclerosis or hardening of arteries due to the presence of plaque can be a cause leading towards heart attacks. One of the causes of atherosclerosis is chronic bacterial and viral infection. As antibiotics are only effective towards bacteria and not viruses it has limited potential to deal with the situation. On the other hand coconut and coconut products have been found to be effective against not only bacteria but viruses as well as other microbes. It works to fight against these pathogens causing chronic infections. Regular intake of coconut and its derivatives and products have a role to play in one way or the other to revert any kind of chronic infections leading to atherosclerosis and consequently towards coronary artery diseases.

Many population studies have resulted in direct correlation between consumption of coconut oil and reduced rates of heart disease and consumption of other oils and fats with increased rates of heart diseases. Same population which had lower risks of heart disease due to high consumption of coconut, coconut oil and its products traditionally started showing signs of increased incidences of these diseases due to increased intake of other types of fats and oils.

Therefore we can conclusively say that increased intake of coconut and its products are directly associated with decreased levels of cardiovascular diseases. They provide hidden powers of protection that need to be understood and studied.

Eating coconut and incorporation of coconut oil in many food items increases the basal metabolic rate. It has also been associated with reduced belly fat which correlates with decreased heart diseases. Fat and fatty acids of coconut oil get easily metabolized and are less likely to get stored in the body in the form of adipose tissues. Fatty acids of coconut oil prefer to get burnt for energy than getting stored. They are also helpful in reducing malnourished.

Stimulation of thermo-genesis by dietary intake of coconut oil in the form of MCT leads to weight loss due to increased energy expenditure. This has been proven through many studies. Increased intake of medium chain fatty triglycerides has been found to have an effect of increased energy expenditure and fat oxidation. According to scientific studies fatty acids from coconut oil are not easily converted to stored body fat but instead get readily utilized by the body.

Coconut oil is directly associated with increased basal metabolic rate leading towards weight loss as weight gain is directly associated with sluggish basal metabolic rate. The presence of lauric acid is invaluable. Lauric acid is also found in mother's milk.

Studies conducted have also revealed that coconut oil helps in reducing belly fat which is otherwise difficult to reduce and is beneficial in prevention and treatment of obesity and overweight.

Coconut Oil For Healthy Skin And Hair.

Coconut oil helps in providing best nourishment needed for having healthy hair and skin. It keeps the renewal process at peak and provides protection from varying atmospheric conditions. It improves the luster of hair by giving them more shine and making them more soft, smooth and silky. It also acts like a natural conditioner and moisturizer that keep dandruff at bay.

Massaging your hair once or twice a week has been found to be helpful in relieving mental stress as well. The same good results have been reported for massaging this oil on face, ears and neck. Our head and face are directly related to our senses and mental capabilities. In addition to having great benefits through internal ingestion it is well qualified to possess hidden secrets of healing power through outer application. Coconut and coconut oil can be called a great natural gift to humanity.

Coconut oil improves skin texture, clears complexion and brightens radiance. It gets easily absorbed by the skin and removes any dryness and makes it soft and healthy. It is usually suitable for all kinds of complexion and skin types. Solidified coconut can be melted through hot water bath in cold climatic conditions as well as could be used in the solid form. The presence of fat soluble vitamins and its fatty acid combination have been tried and tested to provide natural source of nourishment to the skin and hair.

Massaging the head with coconut oil few hours before shampooing can have remarkable results. Even better results can be achieved by leaving it overnight for its soothing effects on brain. Precautionary measures needed to be taken if you want to avoid any kind of undesirable stains and spots on your pillows. You may protect it by covering it with an old shirt or towel.

When using coconut oil on your face you do not have to be careful about avoiding the eye area as it is a natural source and does not possess any kind of harmful effects on any part of the body. With artificial and synthetic creams and lotion

help coconut to regain its lost glory. Many consumers remained deprived of its natural properties and making best use of it in their daily lives.

Since nearly last four decades researchers have known the anti-viral, anti-bacterial and anti-protozoa properties of lauric acid and mono-laurin resulting in more than twenty research papers and numerous patents. A larger group of scientists, clinician and nutritionists have been largely unaware of the full potentials of coconut and coconut oil and many properties of providing diet therapy and various healing factors.

People have started to learn more about it recently. Mono-glycerides and derivatives of medium chain fatty acids can have adverse effects on many micro-organisms e. g. bacteria, fungi, yeast, viruses, etc. Structure of lipids helps in determining its anti-infective actions and mono-glycerides being active while triglycerides are inactive. Myristic acid and capric acid present in coconut oil have lower anti- virus actions than lauric acid which has greater anti-virus action.

Lauric acid is saturated and found in abundance in coconut oil.

Fatty acids and mono-glycerides produce their inactivating and killing effect by lysing the plasma membrane. Mono-laurin solubilize the lipids and phospholipids in the envelope of viruses and disintegrates the viral envelop. The lipid membrane of the viruses is being disrupted by the action of medium chain saturated fatty acids and their derivatives. HIV, herpes virus, measles virus and vesicular stomatitis virus are some of the viruses that could be inactivated by these lipids.

These fatty acids and their derivatives are totally non-toxic to human due to being a natural substance. Lauric acid is one of the best inactivating fatty acids and its derivative mono-glycerides is even better. Mono-laurin does not affect the good type gut bacteria but only attacks the pathogenic ones. Mono-laurin has the capacity to inactivate many pathogenic bacteria including Listeria mono-cytogenes, Staphylococcus aureus, Streptococcus agalactiae,

Streptococci- groups A, F, and G, some gram negative organisms and some gram positive organisms.

Alternative Uses of Coconut and Coconut Oil

Besides dietary and medicinal uses there are various other industrial uses of coconut, coconut oil and its derivatives. A coconut palm tree is supposed to carry more than thousand uses. An eye for innovation is still needed to look for many undiscovered hidden treasures in it. Due to its versatility it has been used for various purposes from building material to jet fuel. It is also being incorporated to produce many cosmetic items.

It has various industrial uses e. g. used in synthesis and production of creams, lotions, detergents, soaps, toothpaste, biofuel, lubricants, deodorants, shampoo, motor oil, bio diesel fuel, engine lubricant, lamp fuel, wood polish, conditioner for wood cutting board, rust inhibitor, bronze polish, plastic, grease, resins, solvents, etc. It is also being used as natural after shave lotion.

It has also been used to power diesel as well as petrol engines as alternative oil and did not cause any problem to the engine. This alternative source of oil has also proved to be environment friendly.

Acid derivatives of coconut oil can also be used as natural herbicide.

Coconut oil is also being used as fuel to generate electricity.

It can be used as a cleanser to clean hands and brush after painting.

Treatment of Ailments

Coconut oil helps in the treatment of many common ailments like cold and flu by acting as a natural anti biotic. It is also known to cure many ailments efficiently due to its typical healing and health giving natural properties. It is a natural medicine with no side effects. It helps in providing sustenance with improved satiety and better metabolism.

It kills or expels lice, giardia, tapeworm and parasites. It provides quick bursts of energy, increases endurance and improves physical activity. It lessens problems associated with cystic fibrosis, etc. It also helps in preventing tooth decay and aids in immune system, prevents liver and kidney diseases, dissolves kidney stones, protects against bladder infection, provides protection against degenerative diseases and premature aging.

It is also beneficial in Alzheimer's disease in which the brain cells are unable to utilize the energy of glucose, therefore they need ketone bodies as an alternative source of energy to function properly. MCT oil a coconut derivative helps in furnishing constant amount of ketones without fasting or ketosis.

Gastro- Esophageal Reflux Disease commonly known as GERD is caused by Helico Pylori Bacteria inhibits the stomach and the esophagus and causes excessive production of hydrochloric acid or gastric juice. This can be painful and can lead to gastritis, ulcers and rarely gastric cancer. Coconut oil works as a natural antibiotic and kills the acid forming bacteria naturally. Fatty acids present in coconut oil kills H. Pylori due to being highly anti- bacterial.

It is also known to improve blood sugar level and risks associated with diabetes. Many symptoms associated with Crohn's disease can also be relieved. Reduces many symptoms associated with gall bladder disease, pancreatitis, hemorrhoids, etc.

In order to summarize coconut and many of coconut derivatives have numerous health and industrial uses. It being a natural source does not pose any kind of adverse health effects. It has much dietary and medicinal therapeutic value. In many food items it can be added in place of other sources of fats for its many beneficial effects and uses. I can also be consumed raw to boast energy and to provide protection against many infections and common ailments. Beside internal benefits it has been known for centuries to possess various outer application benefits.

It provides nourishment to the skin, hair and nails. It is a best type of replacement for artificial and synthetic lotions and cream. It does not possess any kind of synthetic compounds therefore do not possess any kind of health risks. It helps in providing protection against many disease causing germs and bacteria and helps to recover from many diseases by enhancing natural defense mechanism and improving immunity. It helps in increasing the basal metabolic rate and therefore is beneficial in reducing weight and prevention of obesity. It is excellent baby massage oil and can also be used to combat diaper rash.

Its various unusual properties lie in its fat content and the types of fatty acids it possess. Three main types of fatty acids found in coconut and its oil include lauric acid, capric acid and myristic acid. It is a natural saturated fat and therefore in cold climate gets solidified at room temperature. It has pleasant aroma and flavor. It does not get rancid

easily and have long shelf life. It is mostly white in color with wax like texture.

For centuries people living around the world have known to benefit from it in one way or the other. The wood of the tree is also being used to construct houses. Its typical viscosity, melting point, smoking point and chemical content vary it from the rest. Every part of the tree is a blessing in its own sense and being utilized in one way or the other. It has also been tested positively as jet fuel.

According to many studies coconut and coconut oil does not lead to high serum cholesterol level. It is also not a cause for high coronary heart disease. Coconut oil can be used in a variety of ways in the cookery. Baking can be done using this oil instead of other types of fats and oils. It can also be used to pop popcorns and in the making of chocolates.

Coconut oil contains 91 % of saturated fatty acids, 6 % of mono unsaturated fatty acids and 3 % of polyunsaturated fatty acids. It has a smoking temperature of 35 degrees Fahrenheit.

Coconut oil and all derivatives or fractions of coconut oil are beneficial for one reason or the other. Medium chain triglycerides commonly known as MCT oil have many medical applications.

2.5 % of the total world plant oil production comes through coconut oil. Virgin coconut oil VCO is produced by not altering the oil obtained from mature fresh coconut kernel.

Serving size of coconut oil is 100gm which furnishes around 862 calories. It has been used successfully as a diesel engine fuel and can also supply fuel for electricity generation. Philippines is currently using coconut as a fuel for transportation. It has also been used as an engine lubricant. Acid derivatives of coconut oil can be used as a natural herbicide.

As a natural substance it has been known to extend youth. Coconut oil kills disease producing germs and helps in curing many skin, nail and hair problems. It supports the function of thyroid. It also helps in improving blood pressure. It gives strength to bones by helping in better calcium absorption, provides better diabetic control, and prevents cancer.

Coconut can either be eaten raw or can be incorporated into many dishes. It is biodegradable, is light in color and has pleasant flavor and aroma.

Coconut is especially beneficial for skin and many skin diseases. It makes it soft, gives radiance, shine and glow and protects it from heat and climatic conditions. It gets easily absorbed by the skin and helps in improving its color and texture.

It can also be used in oil lamps and the flame does not leave smoke. It is also used in the manufacture of soaps, liquid soaps, shampoo, shaving creams and many cosmetics. It does not contain cholesterol as it is a plant source and it contains vitamin E. It is also used in the manufacture of baby foods.

Coconut oil is made up of medium chain fatty acids or medium chain triglycerides and can easily be burnt to furnish energy. It is stable, is resistant to oxidation and contain low amount of polyunsaturated fatty acids when consumed along with its kernel helps in reducing total serum cholesterol.

It also helps in the absorption of vitamins, minerals and amino acids. Medium and short chain fatty acids containing less than 12 carbon atoms contribute to more than 70 % of the saturated fatty acids found in coconut oil.

Coconut oil is a natural saturated fat from plant which does not possess same risk factors as animal saturated fatty acids. Naturally occurring coconut oil do not possess trans-fatty acids.

It improves insulin efficiency, furnishes quick energy and do not get stored as adipose tissues easily. It also acts like anti parasitic effects, helps in digestion, improves bowel movement and regulates hormones. It also helps in building cells, provides protection from wrinkles and memory loss. Coconut oil helps in retaining youth for a longer period of time.

Coconut water is 100 % sterile and pure. It has highest concentration of naturally occurring electrolytes therefore it is an excellent source of re hydration. It helps the skin to get naturally get rid of the dangerous toxins and helps it to stay smooth, healthy and younger looking for a longer period of time.

It also provides protection against dental cavities and chewing one inch square piece of coconut meat on daily basis helps in keeping the teeth and gums strong.

Coconut oil contains high concentration of short chain and medium chain fatty acids which are necessary for good health. Due to coconuts high fiber content it can add good amount of fiber if added to a diet. It has low glycemic index and helps in maintaining blood glucose level. It reduces cravings for sweets and provides satiety for a longer period of time.

It is a quick source of energy, does not contain trans-fats, is gluten free, hypoallergenic, antibacterial, anti-viral, anti-fungal, and anti-parasitic and supports immune system, healing of wounds and speeds up recovery. It has natural property to work as anti-ulcer, anti-inflammatory, fever reducing and analgesic.

It also possesses brain boosting, fat burning and belly fat reducing property. Approximately one thousand mature coconuts weigh around 1440 kilograms and yield around 70 liter coconut oil and 370g coconut powder. In fractionated coconut oil, a fraction of the whole oil is separated for a variety of uses. Different medium chain fatty acids are separated e. g. lauric acid and capric acid. Lauric acid is a 12 carbon chain fatty acid and is separated for many industrial and medical uses. Capric acid is also fractionated for various different uses e. g. for different diets, medical use, cosmetics and fragrances.

The roots of coconut are beneficial for medicinal use. Its trunk is used to make houses, decorative items, furniture, etc. Coconut leaves can be used to produce high quality natural goods e. g. brooms, paper, hats, mats, fruit trays, hand fans, decorative items, lamp shades, bags, etc.

Flowers, seeds and roots of coconut are used to prepare creams, infusions and pastes for medicinal purposes. Fruit juice is mixed with rice flour and heated and is applied to gangrenous ulcers and skin boils. Fermented juice is being taken as a laxative. The roots are used as an infusion for sore throat gargles. Seeds of coconut are used to treat skin and nasal ulcers.

Coconut oil is applied to scalp to encourage new hair growth and to prevent premature graying. Coconut water mixed with olive oil can be used to get rid of intestinal parasites. It helps in soothing ear ache when mixed with garlic oil and olive oil. Coconut oil supports and repair tissues and reduces muscle and joint inflammation.

Frequently Asked Questions

Q. 1. Is coconut oil a saturated fat?

A. 1. Yes, coconut oil is a saturated fat.

Q. 2. Is it bad for heart?

A. 2. Virgin coconut oil is not bad for the heart. Try to avoid all sorts of hydrogenated fats as they contain trans-fatty acids which can be harmful for the health of the heart.

Q. 3. Is eating coconut, coconut cream and milk as beneficial as coconut oil?

A. 3. Eating whole coconut is even more beneficial due to the presence of fiber and other content.

Q. 4. Can I drink coconut oil as a supplement?

A. 4. Yes, you can consume 1-2 tsp. of coconut oil twice or thrice a day.

Q. 5. Can coconut oil protect me from various diseases?

A. 5. Yes coconut oil has a unique quality of providing protection against various diseases. It works like a natural anti-biotic without having any side effects.

Q. 6. Can it reduce weight?

A. 6. Use it instead of other oils as it helps in increasing basal metabolic rate. Yes it will help in reducing weight especially belly fat.

Q. 7. Can it be used as a skin moisturizer?

A. 7. Yes it can be used as a skin moisturizer and especially good for dry flaky skin.

Q. 8. Can it be used as oil for hair massage?

Q. 8. It is excellent oil for hair massage. It helps in reducing mental stress and depression. It also helps in increasing mental alertness and reducing dandruff.

Q.9. Does it possess any kind of harmful effects?

A. 9. It is a natural substance and therefore does not possess any kind of harmful effects.

Q. 10. Can it be beneficial in the treatment of dandruff?

A. 10. Yes it helps in the controlling and treatment of dandruff.

Q. 11. Does it increase bad type cholesterol?

A. 11.   No it does not increase bad type cholesterol.

Q. 12. Can it help in reducing seizure attacks?

A. 12. Yes it is known to reduce seizure attacks.

Q. 13. Can it work as a natural herbicide?

A. 13. Yes it can work as a natural herbicide.

Q. 14. Does coconut oil possess therapeutic value?

A. 14. Yes it does possess therapeutic value.

Q. 15. Can it be used as a diesel engine fuel?

A. 15. Yes it can be used as a diesel engine fuel.

4. <u>HEALTH, HEALING AND BEAUTY BENEFITS OF APPLE CIDER VINEGAR</u>

Apple cider vinegar also known as cider vinegar or ACV is a pale to amber color vinegar and is made from apple or cider. It is easy and quite inexpensive to make good quality organic, un-filtered and un-pasteurized apple cider vinegar at home level. Fermentation time will depend on the method chosen for making it. In one method the peels, cores and scraps are used. In the second method whole apples may be used.

Using the scraps peels and core method is beneficial in a way that allows you to enjoy your apple as well as utilize the waste to prepare high quality apple cider vinegar. It takes around two months for the apple cider vinegar to ferment from scraps and around six months from whole apples.

For centuries vinegars of many types have been used for many different purposes e. g. marinades, food preservatives, chutneys, salad dressings, meat tenderizer, cleaning, weed controlling, polishing, providing therapy for many ailments, as anti-septic, etc.

Recently apple cider vinegar has started regaining popularity as health supplement and health tonic. Few studies have suggested it to be beneficial in various conditions such as diabetes, obesity, hypertension, heart diseases, fighting infections, helping in digestion, increasing in food satiety value, relieving leg cramps, lowering serum cholesterol level, fighting bad breath, reducing chronic fatigue, reducing swelling,

whitening teeth, killing foot fungus, fighting yeast infection, reducing heart burn, and so on.

Besides having many oral health benefits it has been well known to provide a wide variety of topical application functions and much beauty usage. It can be used as a facial toner, hair rinse, facial mask, bath soak, foot soak, sunburn treatment, age spot removal, deodorant, helps in getting rid of acne, relieves arthritis pain, use as a mouth wash, and so on.

The main contents of vinegar is acetic acid but it may contain other acids and vitamins, minerals, pectin (a soluble fiber), and amino acids, etc. All claims for its highly beneficial effects for all sorts of ailments are not proven through studies but many have ended in conclusion that it might have the potential for many unknown benefits. Besides acetic acid it also contains lactic acid, malic acid and citric acid.

Still few studies suggest that many claims made through experience of generations needed more in depth study to understand and fully utilize the unknown factual benefits hidden and the reasons behind its working. How it actually works inside a human body to benefit it needs better understanding through studies.

For commercial synthesis apples may be crushed to squeeze out the juice. Bacteria and yeast may be added to encourage alcoholic fermentation and its process. Sugar present in apples is turned into alcohol in this way. In the second half of the fermentation process, alcohol gets converted into vinegar by the action of bacteria called acetobacter which helps in the formation of acetic acid. Malic acid and acetic acid gives vinegar its sour taste. Conventional method of its production will need time and patience for the process of fermentation happening naturally. For large commercial production, quick processing methods may be applied to produce huge amounts of it in a short period of time.

There are also several other ways to produce apple cider vinegar on large scale for commercial purposes. Vinegar helps in adding the satiety of foods and a person who consumes it through meals experiences fullness for a longer period of time. It also reduces heart burn and regularizes bowel movement. It is also known to relieve chest congestion and boosts energy. It works as a blood thinner, provides relief from jelly fish sting pain, skin irritation, bug bite and aids in reducing blood pressure.

It provides more satiety of food and this may be a cause behind its association with weight loss besides other causes. According to the studies conducted in relation to vinegar with weight loss, it has been concluded that it might reduce body weight and obesity. More studies are needed to fully understand the working and relationship of it to weight reduction.

Very high intake for a long period of time may lead to hyper-reninemia, hyperkalemia and osteoporosis.

As apple cider vinegar is highly acidic its intake needed to be incorporated through dietary intake instead of isolated intake as direct intake causes skin burn due to it being highly acidic in nature. Even it can have burning effect on skin through outer application if applied in concentration.

More studies are needed in the area to fully understand the benefits of it and to segregate myths with facts in order to find the true value behind. It has been associated with providing natural remedies for many kinds of chronic diseases e. g. acid reflux, acne, constipation, weight loss, control of blood sugar, memory problems, reversing aging, etc.

ACV also acts like blood thinner and may also help in the prevention of high blood pressure. From during the time of Hippocrates it has been considered to be the father of all cures. During the wars it was being used as an antiseptic to treat the wounds. It is known to work as a natural detoxifying agent, providing relief from allergies, balancing the body pH, reducing inflammation and preventing flu.

How to incorporate it in our meals so that we can make the best use of it and ingest it in a way that gives us full potential of its benefits without overdosing it or taking it in isolation. Incorporating it in our meals to bring out the best possible results needs a real challenging situation. It is possible only by giving due consideration towards it and understanding the benefits attached to it by doing so.

Apples being highly nutritious fruit contain a wide variety of vitamins, minerals, amino acids, enzymes, pectin, etc. And in the making of apple cider vinegar apples are the main ingredients. All vinegars do not possess the same kind of natural remedial value as apple cider vinegar does. It also contains many enzymes, microbes and all the bye products produced during the processing.

It helps in purifying and detoxifying many body organs. It assists in oxidizing of blood, neutralizing toxic body substances and pathogenic bacteria, and promotes digestion and elimination process. There are also claims of it helping in the strengthening of the heart and anti-carcinogenic effects on certain types of cancers. Vinegar contains chromium which could have an altering effect on your insulin level.

Vinegar can be made from many fruits, vegetables and grains but apple cider vinegar as the name suggest is made from pulverized apples. No other vinegar possesses the same qualities as ACV. From being used as a folk remedy it has recently gained a more modern approach on its uses and benefits based on studies and researches.

ACV may also interact with medication for diabetes and heart diseases as well as with laxatives and diuretics. Food drug interaction needs to be understood fully by patients utilizing these medications for their treatment before starting on a new remedy.

You can make your own apple cider vinegar at home and can be sure of its quality and purity without having doubts that you might have about all the available commercial brands. Wash apples, dice them and put them in a glass jar. Do not remove peels and core. Fill water in the jar to cover the apples. Cover the jar with a piece of cloth or paper towel so that the oxygen can pass through it. Place the jar in a clean, dry, dark and warm place. Leave it to ferment for at least six months. Keep stirring it once a week for good results. After six months you will observe a layer of scum caused by bacteria on top of it. Filter the content with a cheese cloth. Let it stand for another 4-6 weeks for good results. Cover the jar and refrigerate it for longer storage.

PREVENTS STOMACH PROBLEMS

Apple cider vinegar has a natural bacteria fighting power and may contain magnesium, chlorine, phosphorus, potassium, sulfur, sodium, calcium, iron, copper and fluorine. It has been claimed to provide relief from indigestion problems, stomach churning, pain, acid reflux, constipation, heart burn, neutralizing toxic substances and bacteria, etc.

It can be added during food preparation for its consumption and can be used in moderate amounts on a daily basis to make full use of its therapeutic value and to improve the peristaltic movement of the gut. It is also known to flush out toxic waste from the body which helps in keeping the digestive system in peak condition.

One tea spoon full of it can be added in juices with honey to make a balanced drink. Besides it can also be added in soups, purees, gravies, sauces, salads, marinades and many more.

Pickles, relishes and chutneys prepared from apple cider vinegar could be made a part of each meal to make a better use of it on a daily diet plan.

Use of ACV for health benefits helps in better making use of the natural remedies available which is being avoided and hindered by the pharmacological sector of any given society due to their vested interests strategic view.

For the relief of acid reflux, heart burn and nausea it has been recommended to add it to your drink with honey or in your soup 30 minutes or one hour before your meal. Within three days' time it has been claimed to relieve a person of all these   symptoms.

CALMS DOWN DIGESTION

It helps in increased production of gastric juices and enzymes needed for proper digestion of each food eaten. These enzymes help in the breaking down of the food items into smaller and smaller pieces so that these valuable nutrients could be absorbed by the blood stream during digestion and benefits the body by providing nourishment whenever and where ever needed.

It also helps in increasing the acidity of food which is needed for digestion. Presence of pectin which is a soluble fiber must have a role to play in having a calming effect on digestion and intestinal spasm. Its antibiotic property can help in relieving diarrhea caused by bacteria.

The strong smell and typical strong taste of apple cider vinegar will be a little difficult to handle it in the beginning, but once you get used to it you can make it a regular part of your daily routine. To provide best natural remedies for your overall wellness and to make use of the great beneficial value provided by apple cider vinegar, it needs to be kept handy in your kitchen.

CLEARS NASAL CONGESTION

Apple cider vinegar helps in clearing the nasal congestion by steam inhalation. You may add it to your humidifier for the beneficial results and breathe it in. You may also add a little apple cider vinegar to a bowl and then pour boiling water in it. Start inhaling the steam till the water cools down. Repeating it twice or thrice daily can help you in getting relief from the symptoms in a natural way.

HELPS WITH HICCUPS

Hiccups usually lasts for a few minutes but at times may continue to last for a longer period of time which could be a cause of irritability and discomfort. Many natural remedies could be used to control it at home level before proceeding towards medical intervention or help. One such remedy is the use of apple cider vinegar in a drink to overcome it and to

get relief from it. People have been trying it and have found it to be of substantially beneficial.

Take a cup of warm drinking water, add one tea spoon full of apple cider vinegar and two tea spoons full of honey in it, stir well and consume it sip by sip. If the problem persists for longer period of time than medical help may be advisable.

Hiccup is a repeated involuntary contraction of the diaphragm and in medical terminology is known as singultus or synchronous diaphragmatic flutter (SDF). Usually it is self-limiting and gets resolved without any intervention naturally. Apple cider vinegar can be tried initially as a natural home remedy. If the problem persists and gets chronic, medical attention may be considered.

SOOTHS YOUR SORE THROAT

Symptoms of sore throat can be treated successfully at home level through the use of apple cider vinegar appropriately. As apple cider vinegar has anti-bacterial properties it can help in fighting infections especially the one causing a sore throat. The pH of the tissues gets decreased by the acidity of the vinegar which helps in preventing bacterial growth on the surface. The presence of pre biotic inulin in raw ACV helps in increasing the number of white blood cells and T cells and boosts the immune system.

Consuming apple cider vinegar through a hot beverage and soups and sipping it twice or thrice daily can help in relieving sore throat. Adding a tea spoon full in your hot beverage or soup may help in soothing the symptoms. While resting after its consumption can bring out more beneficial results in shorter period of time.

Do not use apple cider vinegar more than one tea spoon at a time as it is acetic acid and could harm your tooth enamel if taken in excess or in high concentration. Taking one teaspoon full through a food medium is enough to bring out all the beneficial effects needed. Overdosing will not help in any way therefore patience is needed after you have used a natural remedy for your sore throat symptoms.

REDUCES SWELLING IN HANDS AND FEET

Natural home remedies are simple, tried and tested at home level, hassle free, in-expensive and easily approachable. Good use of common sense is needed when deciding upon when to use a simple natural home remedy and when to look for an expert's opinion. Serious medical condition need not be ignored.

In case of chronic medical condition do consult your medical practitioner before you use any kind of home remedy.

Swelling of hand and feet can be caused by fluid retention by the cells and tissues of the body and commonly referred to as edema. Edema can be a cause of pregnancy, PMS, high blood pressure, poor nutrition, menopause, cardiovascular diseases, cirrhosis of liver, kidney disease, swelling of the lymph nodes, etc.

Excessive intake of common salt in the diet may also help in retaining extra water in the body. It can also be caused by lack of potassium. The treatment needed to be based on resolving the underlying cause or causes of extra water inside the body leading to swelling. Apple cider vinegar is a natural home remedy that helps the body to remove extra fluids.

ACV can be consumed as mentioned earlier through a beverage or a soup. Only take a teaspoon full at a time once or twice daily. An apple cider vinegar soak can also benefit. Soak a piece of cloth in undiluted ACV and for at least fifteen minutes keep it wrapped around the swollen area. Another way to treat it is to immerse the affected area into one part ACV mixed with three parts of water. Besides possessing other active ingredients ACV also contain potassium which helps in relieving and treating symptoms of swelling naturally but not to the extent of relieving deficiencies. High potassium food sources needed to be added to avoid and to reverse the effects of deficiency if any.

REDUCES FATIGUE

Chronic fatigue can be a result of imbalanced dietary intake, stress, tension, lack of sleep and rest, dehydration and it can also be a cause of some underlying chronic condition or disease which needed to be investigated.

Release of lactic acid during exercising and prolong stress can cause fatigue. Apple cider vinegar helps in combating this with the help of its unique content of enzymes, potassium, amino acids and other substances. Drinking it through hot beverages and soups may help in relieving the symptoms gradually. Do not try to consume more than what has been recommended earlier. Also look towards the underlying causes of it and try to overcome these by properly eliminating the causes.

RELIEVES LEG CRAMPS

Leg cramps usually is not a serious problem but can be quite irritating and painful. There can be various underlying reasons behind this illness e. g. irregular muscle contraction, dehydration, electrolyte or mineral imbalance, etc. Low potassium level can also be a contributing factor leading towards these cramps especially the nocturnal type which you might be experiencing quite frequently.

Apple cider vinegar may help in overcoming the imbalances. One tea spoon full can be added to warm water with honey and can be taken twice or thrice daily to overcome this situation naturally. In addition to this eating foods that are high in potassium will help in overcoming the deficiency. Good food sources of potassium include banana, dried fruits, avocado, fresh mushrooms, milk and its products, tomatoes, potatoes, white beans, fish, squash, leafy green vegetables, etc.

Sodium in addition to potassium is responsible for maintaining the water balance in a human body. Consuming juices with a pinch of salt added can also help. Increasing your calcium and magnesium intake might also help. You may add a teaspoon full of apple cider vinegar with honey in your cocktail for effective results.

Drinking enough water and fluid is needed if the underlying cause is dehydration. You may also massage the affected area with undiluted ACV. Taking a hot bath and soaking the affected area may too benefit. Looking for the underlying cause and correcting the same will help in getting rid of the problem from its roots.

FIGHTS BAD BREATH

Halitosis or bad breath can be a sign of certain health problems. One of the common causes of it includes dental cavities, improper cleaning, cracked fillings, etc. Eating certain foods can also be a cause but which cannot and should not be avoided for its high nutritive value as these are essential for good health and wellbeing.

It can also be caused by bacteria feeding on food particles trapped in the mouth. Saliva production continuously provide natural cleansing ability and bad breath can also be a cause of xerostomia in which the mouth is dry due to lack of saliva production.

Many underlying diseases can also cause bad breath e. g. chronic bronchitis, constipation, diabetes, respiratory tract infection, liver disease, etc. Artificial and synthetic mouthwash can solve the problem temporarily and can contain substances that may be carcinogenic. Healthier, cheaper and natural substances can be used to overcome the problem without any side effects.

Adding one tea spoon full of each apple cider vinegar and honey to warm water, juice or cocktail and consuming it half an hour before meals can help in overcoming this problem naturally. Gargling after each meal with a diluted solution of ACV and water may also be effective.

It possesses a quality of being natural antibiotic and anti-septic which helps in fighting with these bad breath causing bacteria. It helps in increasing the secretion of saliva which will contribute as a natural cleanser. Good oral hygiene is a must in any case. Drinking too much coffee, sugary drink, alcohol and smoking can easily be avoided without affecting nutrition intake.

FIGHTS YEAST INFECTIONS

The natural acetic acid bacteria present in apple cider vinegar has the capability of fighting against yeast infection caused by Candida Albican. This yeast can cause infection in various parts of a human body e. g. gastric and esophageal lining, skin, mouth, etc. Through natural treatment of apple cider vinegar the growth of yeast is being restricted and hampered by good type bacteria.

The composition of ACV is such that it helps in boosting the body's immune system to fight against such infections. It could be consumed through a beverage, soup or through foods as well as could be applied on the affected areas with the help of a cotton wool or a piece of cloth. Rinsing your body with a diluted solution of vinegar and water for outer infection may also help.

You may need to consult a physician if you are unable to restrain the infection through natural therapy or if the infection seems to be spreading.

KILLS FOOT FUNGUS

A simple home remedy can help in getting relief from nail and toe fungus. ACV naturally possesses anti-fungal properties and it can provide a slow but definite cure for it. You will have to be patient for the result as fungal growth inside a nail is difficult to reach and cure. Other cure from medics may involve medication which every one might not be able to take. Surgical removal of the nail can be another option which many would like to avoid.

Apple cider vinegar could help in treating it naturally by oral intake as well as outer application to the affected area. Low sugar foods must follow this natural remedy. Without surgery or medication you will be able to get rid of it hopefully within a year's time naturally.

CONTROLS BLOOD SUGAR

According to the results of various studies conducted to understand the role of ACV in controlling blood sugar in diabetic patients is quite promising for its health benefits. Vinegar contains chromium which can alter the insulin level so medical advice is needed to be sought before starting to begin with this natural remedy.

If it is used in combination with diet and exercise it can help people with type 2 diabetes which is usually non-insulin dependent. It has been discovered that acetic acid the main constituent of apple cider vinegar inhibits the activity of many enzymes needed for carbohydrates digestion and absorption e. g. amylase, maltase, lactase and sucrase.

In the presence of ACV in the digestive tract a part of ingested sugars and starches will pass through without either getting digested or being absorbed by the blood.

INCREASES WEIGHT LOSS

Apple cider vinegar helps in losing weight by providing more satiety to foods as well as eliminating part of carbohydrates intake without being absorbed by the blood. More significant studies in the area are needed to fully understand the mechanism if any attached to the many claims being made.

LOWERS YOUR CHOLESTEROL

Apples are good source of soluble fiber like pectin. Apple cider vinegar primarily made from apples contains pectin which is a soluble fiber. Soluble fibers help in eliminating the dietary cholesterol instead of it being absorbed by the body by binding with it and getting excreted. It also helps in reducing the synthesis of cholesterol by the liver. Therefore it has been claimed to bring out the result of lowering serum cholesterol if taken in small amounts on daily basis especially through incorporation in meals.

USE AS A HAIR RINSE

Apple cider vinegar has several beauty benefits besides its many health benefits. It has great treatment effects if used as a hair rinse. It helps in the treatment of dandruff, hair loss, balancing scalp pH, removing various product buildup, etc. It also assists in improving the texture of hair and leaves them smooth, soft and shiny. It also aids in preventing split ends, dry scalp, frizz, tangles, etc.

It also assists in maintaining and replenishing the moisture of your hair. If used in combination with baking soda can work as a natural conditioner. The ideal pH for hair is slightly on the acidic side.

Using the shampoos which are alkaline leaves the pH on the higher side. To bring it back to a lower side ACV rinse brings out the best results needed. It adds beauty, bounce and body to your hair naturally.

USE AS A FACIAL MASK

To give a finishing rinse to your face in order to cleanse it, treat it against microbes and to tighten the skin ACV facial mask can be used. It can also be used in combination with other beneficial ingredients e. g. honey. It should be applied over the face and left for treatment for at least 20 minutes. This mask could be used thrice weekly to bring out moisturizing and healing benefits as well as to maintain the pH of your skin. It can also be mixed with clay, or any of your favorite mask base to sooth and treat your skin once fortnightly or whenever needed especially in hot summer season.

TONES YOUR SKIN

Poor skin tone makes it appear uneven and older. Unbalanced dietary intake, over exposure to sunlight and aging can all contribute negatively to skin tone. To improve your skin tone you can utilize the beneficial effects of apple cider vinegar to control oil production, to give smooth texture and appearance to the skin and to clear blemishes.

It being a natural anti biotic also helps in reducing the breakouts caused by bacteria and yeast. Acids also help your skin to have more elasticity and keep it youthful for a longer period of time. As ACV is a natural product you do not have to worry about the chemical composition and harsh effects due to being synthetic.

It also improves blood circulation towards skin and gives it natural life and lift needed. To make a good toner, add equal amount of water and ACV in a bottle. Add few drops of your favorite oil and the toner is ready for application. Use it after washing your face by taking a little in your palm and applying it over your face. Repeat it 3 - 4 times weekly for good results.

USE AS A BATH SOAK

Apple cider vinegar bath soak can eliminate or reduce discomfort caused by sunburn. Add one cup of ACV to you bath and soak for at least 10 minutes to get relief from this discomfort. In order to recover from infection and inflammation this simple natural remedy will be beneficial. Also to detoxify your body you may avail the ACV bath soak. ACV can be used for detoxifying effects needed alone or in combination with other natural compounds.

It can be used for pain relief, to increase immunity, detoxification, sunburn, pain relief, athlete's foot, UTI, arthritis, etc. It also helps in maintaining the pH of the body and lowering stress related hormones. One cup of raw, unprocessed, organic apple cider vinegar can be added into warm bath. Half an hour of soaking the body in this solution will help in bringing out balancing changes needed.

WHITENS YOUR TEETH

Gargling with ACV in the morning may help in removing stains on teeth, whitens it and kills bacteria. Brush your teeth after gargling. For good result use it consistently for at least one whole month as nicotine and coffee stains are stubborn and difficult to remove.

Olive oil together with apple cider vinegar can be used as an alternative to a tooth paste for brushing your teeth for good results. ACV can also be used in isolation for the beneficial effects but do not use in excess or in saturation as it can damage the tooth enamel.

Besides using it as mouth wash or a tooth paste it needed to be taken orally through meals in a variety of ways to bring out best results. Many food items which are also helpful in whitening the teeth naturally include lemons, oranges, strawberries, carrots, broccoli, etc.

USE AS A FOOT SOAK

Apple cider vinegar can be used as a foot soak to get relief from foot odor, toe fungus, athletes foot, etc. It also helps in softening and soothing of dry skin and cracked heels. ACV foot soak can be used in many foot problems and conditions e. g. fatigued foot, warts, calluses, regular foot cure, etc.

Patients who are suffering from chronic diseases need to first consult their physician before starting on this home remedy especially people who have diabetes.

USE TO TREAT SUN BURN

Apple cider vinegar works well to treat and prevent sunburn by helping the skin to combat inflammation caused by it. To treat sunburn make use of diluted apple cider vinegar solution through a piece of cloth on the affected areas, let it dry and then spread a little amount of your favorite oil on it.

Follow this for a few days till it all heals up naturally. Sun burn can be quite discomforting caused due to excessive exposure to sunlight and may start showing signs within few hours which could range from mild to severe.

In severe condition medical intervention may be needed. It is better to avoid exposing skin to direct sunlight to prevent it to occur. Many synthetic sun blocks may contain chemical substances that can result in exposing your body to unnatural substances which may be a contributing factor in causing severe skin diseases and disorders.

GET RID OF AGE SPOTS

Application of apple cider vinegar on age spots with a piece of cloth or cotton helps in combating these naturally. Age spots are flat, brown or yellow discoloration of the skin and can occur on the hands, neck and face. These can be a cause of sun damage, improper liver function, nutrient deficiency, chronic constipation, lack of sleep, dehydration, lack of dietary intake of antioxidants, etc.

ACV can be applied in the diluted form as well as with many other combinations for better result. It can be used in combination with onion juice, sandal powder, rose water or olive oil.

NATURAL DEODORANT

After getting aware of all the harmful effects caused by much marketed and advertised varieties of deodorants and antiperspirant available in all the beautiful packaging, colors and shiny containers, one begins to start wondering about the alternatives and natural substitutes available.

Switching over to these natural remedies might need will power and tactics of simplifying through simple means instead of complicating it through synthetic means. Results of the uses of all sorts of synthetic living have started to show negative signs from all angles which could and should easily be avoided.

Many irreversible health damages could happen and therefore prevention is better than cure. Replacing all your artificial synthetic products with natural simple ones needs understanding of how each one works well. Apply diluted apple cider vinegar in place of synthetic deodorant for better overall results.

GET RID OF ACNE

The presence of acids in apple cider vinegar aids in ex foliating the dead cells, removing oil and fighting bacteria. Dab a piece of cloth in half strength solution of apple cider vinegar and water and apply it over your face giving special attention to the affected areas.

Green tea or your favorite oil can be added to get rid of the strong smell of apple cider vinegar. Having natural antibiotic properties it may help in killing bacteria causing this problem. It also helps in restoring the pH of our skin. How much time is needed for curing this will differ with each individual case.

Pure unfiltered apple cider vinegar can be used for this purpose. If you find the smell to be intolerable then apply only to the affected areas.

GET RID OF WARTS

Apple cider vinegar has been found to be successful in removing warts by people who have tried this home remedy. Warts are common dermatological problem which could be treated easily at home level with very low cost and without any side effects through AC V's proper application.

Warts are caused by viruses entering through cuts and breaks in the skin. Before going to bed soak a piece of cotton wool in ACV and keep over the wart and fasten it with Band-Aid. In the morning replace the old piece of cotton and Band-Aid with a fresh one. If it bothers you in the day time then only keep it at night time.

Keep repeating this for at least one week so that the chances of it re-appearing diminish and the problem gets solved from the roots.

RELIEVES ARTHRITIS PAIN

Topical application of apple cider vinegar mixed with olive oil and coconut oil can work wonders to relieve the pain of joints. Before going to sleep at night massage the effected painful areas of joint with this solution for at least ten to fifteen minutes. You can also apply heat after massage by resting the affected area on hot water bottle. Resting and sleeping is also very important.

Individual cases of arthritis may vary from each other. There are different forms of arthritis e. g. juvenile arthritis, osteoarthritis, rheumatoid arthritis, septic arthritis, psoriatic arthritis, etc. Osteoarthritis is the most common form which is a degenerative disease of joints. Causes of osteoarthritis may involve age, infection of joints or it may be a result of trauma.

Major complaints may include persistent localized joint pain. It occurs due to inflammation around the joint and various other reasons. Apple cider vinegar benefits can also be availed to help reduce symptoms associated with joint pain by incorporating it through salads and dietary intake.

All varieties of fruits and vegetables are highly recommended for these patients to overcome the underlying causes. Best uses of fruits and vegetables which could be consumed in raw form needed to be made. Reducing weight by the intake of low calories and highly nutritious diet is needed. Increasing activity to tolerable degree is advisable to keep the joints in good working condition and to reduce weight if needed.

HELPS IN KILLING CANCER CELLS

Studies done to understand the role of apple cider vinegar to treat cancer patients have revealed certain facts that may be helpful in killing cancer cells or regressing their growth. But still no conclusive hypothesis is available currently to suggest any fact with guarantee.

ACV is acidic in nature but once inside the body it promotes the body towards increased alkalinity which is needed to treat cancer.

USE AS A MOUTH WASH

Apple cider vinegar in diluted form can be used as a mouthwash to combat bad breath as well as to provide anti septic properties once daily to help prevent cavities and infection and to cleanse your mouth.

Artificial and synthetic mouthwash contains many chemicals which have been found to be carcinogenic. In order to avoid these chemicals as they leave their residue in mouth, good use of better natural alternatives is needed.

After studying the benefits of apple cider vinegar at length we come to a solid conclusion that it needed to be made a part of dietary intake in whatever way it is feasible on a daily basis. It can be incorporated in a variety of ways while cooking and preparing meals for example, salads, soups, beverages, marinating of entree, casseroles, gravies, curries, breads, biscuits, etc.

Innovative ideas could be applied to create great recipes of interest and individual liking. People who like sour flavor would not find it hard to use it and apply it in their cookery methods and creations. Chinese cookery methods make high use of vinegar in their foods. Anyone who is fond of eating Chinese cuisine would also not find it difficult.

Vinegar also acts like a meat tenderizer. While cooking mutton, lamb or beef you may marinate the meat in apple cider vinegar for at least 3-4 hours before cooking to let the meat absorb its good sour flavor as well as tenderize it for easy cooking and also helping in lessening the time needed for meat to get tender. If you prepare it one day before and keep it refrigerated, it could bring out really good results.

Pickles, relishes and chutneys could easily be prepared at home level using apple cider vinegar and a variety of vegetables of individual likings and disliking. It need not be consumed in large amount as it is pure acid and needed to be used sparingly but regularly.

Besides meals it has many other beneficial uses from being as a house cleanser to a body cleanser. It has numerous other health and healing benefits. These simple home remedies helps in bringing simple ways and methods of doing things which helps in making living easier and worthy. In today's life of artificiality and modernization, people had been leaving behind the wisdom of the wise which need not be ignored or forgotten.

After we have become fully aware of the dangers of consuming synthetic chemicals in the form of medication even for simple health problems which could easily be resolved by good rest, sleep, eating pattern and living style. We have seen the results of the side effects these are causing not just to one person, or family, or community but in the global form.

People need to realize the importance of avoiding chemicals as much in their lives as possible not only in diet but all around their lives. Natural therapies and home remedies could wisely be applied as much as possible. Simple life makes it easier and even much cheaper with immeasurable benefits. The need only lies in realization of it and working towards it.

There are a wide variety of topical benefits attached with apple cider vinegar. These benefits may include soaking, massaging, gargling, brushing, toning, cleansing, disinfecting, treating, rinsing, etc. It can also be used with other natural substances to improve or increase its potency. Just be sure not to use any products for experimentation which might lead to many kinds of problematic situations.

Get well aware and use combinations that have been tried and tested. If you feel confident that you're created therapy works for you then do share it with others so that other people get well aware of it too. Responsible behavior towards this is needed as each ones wellbeing is others responsibility.

Do not use apple cider vinegar in concentration as it is quite potent, strong and harsh. Do use a base for some kind of dilution. Also do not be an extremist when it comes to dietary intake. Quick fixes by over dosing will only help in ruining your health and affecting it negatively. Patience is needed, and only thinks of it as a part of medication instead of part of a diet. As you are careful about not taking medications in excess so think the same way with ACV as it is no less than a medication when it comes to over dosing.

Think about it when in concentrated form it works like a meat tenderizer and when it goes inside your body in that saturated form what will happen inside. So never ever use it in saturation but use it as a salad dressing, flavor enhancer, meat tenderizer, and in many different ways in moderation that allows you to consume it as a part of meal and incorporated in your meal in small amounts. Concentrated forms of it might have a damaging effect on your tooth enamel, tissues and cells of your body and many unknown problems.

Use in concentrated form for outer application only as an anti-septic or to fight fungal growth and to treat warts. It can also be used as a treatment for insect bite, to reduce cellulite, fight infections, ease pain, and fade bruises, sooth bug bite and to relieve inflammation.

It is a very affordable and natural type of deodorant. Synthetic deodorants and antiperspirants act by blocking the sweating ability. Sweating is a natural body process to get rid of the toxins present inside. In this way it hinders the body's capability to detoxify. ACV gets absorbed and it helps in neutralizing the body perspiration odor.

ACV is acidic but once inside the body it promotes the body towards increased alkalinity which is a good sign for our health. It is also known to dissolve kidney stones. The best known fact about apple cider vinegar is its natural anti biotic properties and it is well known to possess anti-bacterial, anti-viral and anti-fungal properties.

ACV is also known to help relieve gout, gum infection, candida infection, sinus infection, ear infection, rheumatism, etc. It reacts positively with body toxins and helps in getting relief from them. But one thing is certain that no doubt it does possess numeral benefits to health and healing but cannot be a source of nourishment. People have been making it a part of food source which it cannot be. A very simple test at home level can prove it. Start boiling your ACV and evaporate all the water content of it. The total substance left in the end as residue is all the nourishment that it contains. Which you can see is negligible to the amount of nourishment that you need to take to stay healthy and well nourished. So please do not use it as a source of nourishment.

If you need potassium do look towards foods rich in potassium instead of believing ACV to overcome the deficiencies. It does contain a variety of nutrients but in insignificant quantity. Instead of calling it a tonic it needed to be called an antibiotic. Its antibiotic properties are much stronger and potent especially the outer application which cannot and should not be ignored.

Apple cider vinegar does not possess cure for all diseases. And the ones it has been promoted for do not   possess solid scientific backing. Tried and tested by many as a successful home remedy for centuries it does not possess any obvious harmful effects known to us till now. Therefore trying it does not feature any side effects associated with it. Obviously over emphasizing its importance for all cures will lead to misguidance and various health risk factors.

 It has been an ingredient of a part of cookery, medicine, beauty care, and many more. People have been mesmerized by much antibiotic

potency it contains. Its true value need to be known and there is only one way of doing so is by finding facts about it through scientific research studies. Until this is done we know that it is only a natural substance and could be taken in moderation regularly without worrying about the side effects and negative cost to our health and wellbeing.

5. *HEALTH AND HEALING POWER   OF MEDITERRANEAN DIET*

A 'Mediterranean Diet' or 'Mediterranean Cuisine' is based on the customary or habitual dietary consumption pattern having typical features related to various cultures and civilizations scattered around and adjacent to Mediterranean Sea. A great variety of various cultures living with many historical connections in the region has led to many common and similar elements leading to the development of 'Mediterranean Cuisine' or 'Mediterranean Diet'.

This diet has been associated with many health giving factors. It is considered to be beneficial for over-all health, well-being and increased life expectancy. Several population studies have revealed its importance which was surfaced during 1050's. It recently started gaining recognition due to its good composition of healthy foods which makes good use of some of the most health giving foods. It has been considered to provide much health giving factors and reducing chances of developing various diseases and increasing life expectancy.

Although this diet has been prevalent in this part of the world for many centuries, its true value and importance could not be understood well before. It has been gaining popularity and interest in many other parts of the world due to its healthy composition and balance which helps in giving protection from various food items which have been affecting negatively to over-all health while giving rise to many chronic diseases.

Generally this diet makes the best use of plant sources of foods e. g. vegetables, fruits, nuts, seeds, whole grains and beans. It provides an abundant amount of fish and olive oil. Red meat and sweets are consumed occasionally. Red wine is taken customary during meal times.

Togetherness and meal sharing is habitual and being encouraged and meal time is an enjoyment, happy and fun time for all. Increasing physical activity and exercising is also emphasized and is a typical pattern of life of people living in this region of the world. It is a heart friendly diet which is quite evident through studies. It helps in lowering serum cholesterol level, blood pressure, incidence of cancer and several chronic diseases. It has also been revealed to suggest that it might also be helpful in decreasing our chances of having Alzheimer's, osteoporosis, depression and diabetes. Studies have also suggested it to be beneficial in reducing overall body weight if used for more than six months besides increasing physical activity and reducing overall intake of calories. It has been considered to show better results than a low fat diet.

It stresses on utilizing plant sources of foods while using yogurt, eggs and poultry to a lesser extent. At least twice a week, intake of fish and seafood is being encouraged. All fat sources come through good sources e. g. olives, olive oil, extra virgin olive oil, nuts seeds, avocado, etc. instead of using butter and margarine. Various beneficial herbs and spices are used to improve and enhance the flavor of food while salt is used sparingly. Red wine is being consumed in moderation, usually a glass for ladies and one or two for gents. But drinking water is being encouraged for more beneficial health benefits.

Fruits usually replace desserts and snacks and in this way this diet discourages more usage of simple sugars and saturated fat consumption which is being associated with many ailments and chronic diseases. Red meat and dessert are usually consumed occasionally. This type of diet is being consumed by many for its many beneficial health giving factors as well as good taste. One can easily learn the techniques to apply and use for great health and taste benefits by experimentation and learning in a variety of ways. Many methods e. g. grilling, broiling, baking, etc. could be used to prepare these.

To make the best use of this diet for long term use, plan your cooking and shopping in advance. Look and learn from many available recipes and make best use of these for great health benefits. Its main features include utilization of simple means of essential food items in simple ways to reap out the best outcome by increased health benefits.

In this, nuts could be replaced for snacks which are rich in saturated fats and simple sugars helps in benefiting in relieving from many disease causing factors. Having a handful of humble nuts and pita with hummus means a good way of following a 'Mediterranean Diet'. Instead of making use of many frozen, canned, processed and partially prepared food items, it makes best use of mostly fresh supplies of foods which helps in increasing its purity level.

In this way people are more capable of protecting themselves from many harmful effects of various food additives, preservatives, synthetic chemical substances and artificial colors. Food is being consumed in a wholesome manner which allows you to be totally sure of the quality of contents and food items used. It helps in minimizing your chances of eating lots of chemicals and processed food stuff.

Processing of foods also effects negatively to the nutrient content of foods. This needed to be discouraged all together for better health and improved quality.

It can be called an adaptive version of traditional dietary intake of people living in regions bordering Mediterranean Sea. Countries bordering Mediterranean Sea have deep and rich history and this is a place where many civilizations flourished and left their marks behind e. g. Phoenicia, Sicily, Rome and Carthage.

Mediterranean people are inhabitants of countries located in this region. These people belong to the Caucasoid race and are characterized by slender built and dark complexion. Geographically speaking, the climate is characterized by hot summers and relatively warm winter. Rainfall mostly occurs during the winter season.

Surrounded and situated completely or nearly in the middle of landmass or dry land, the region started to be known as 'Mediterranean' meaning in the middle of land. Mediterranean Sea is the largest inland sea between Asia, Africa and Europe. Many countries, islands and areas have specific importance due to their location and various factors associated with this.

Countries from Europe which are part of this region include Spain, Gibraltar, France, Monaco, Italy, Malta, Croatia, Bosnia Herzegovina, Slovenia, Montenegro, Albania, Crete, Greece and Turkey. Countries which are located within Asia and are part of this region include Syria, Lebanon, Palestine and Israel. Countries which belong to Africa but are considered to be part of this region include Egypt, Libya, Tunisia, Algeria and Morocco.

Historically, this region has been associated with folk story of Prophet Jonah, who got swallowed alive by a huge whale, who after few days found himself alive by the sea-side. All these countries and territories and many colonies and islands belong to and show remarkable characteristic typical features of this region.

Historically speaking, there have been many similarities in culture and traditions of neighboring countries while cultural clashes of civilizations which have been impacting and giving new dimensions to various cultural norms. It is difficult to dispute the geographical unity which has seen one of the oldest civilizations of mankind.

Prosperity and destruction, peace and war have all been part as well as development of many important ports and cities. The importance of the history of this region is due to the location of Mediterranean Sea where many cultures and societies integrated with each other while many preferred to flourish in isolation.

For culinary purpose, we can divide this region into main countries showing typical features of this diet which include Morocco, Egypt, Greece, Israel, Lebanon, Syria, Turkey, Italy, France and Spain. Wine and dine are used for social purposes in many areas while herbs and spices are consumed in many other areas. Wine and herbs are common in the Central and Southern Europe Cuisine, while bold use of spices is common in North African Cuisine.

The use of a wide variety of fresh foods is helpful in making this diet very appealing to the eye due to its rich color, and the use of a wide variety of health giving herbs and spices enhances the aroma and flavor of food.

People who are interested in living with great harmony with nature would love to support the benefits acquired through the traditional offering of rich aroma and beautiful natural colors of a wide variety of foods that need to be consumed in a more natural and fresher manner.

The basic idea behind adhering to this diet is not how you consume it through various cooking procedures, methods or recipes, but the main content of its composition and over-all approach towards making the right kind of choices based on facts revealed through population studies. One needs to know how to combine foods in a manner that will help in leading towards more beneficial aspects for a longer period of time. Besides giving clues to many beneficial factors, it also emphasizes in restricting certain foods to lessen our chances of developing many chronic diseases and mortality and morbidity rates.

The Mediterranean basin has been recalled by many historians as 'the cradle of society' due to having geographical borders where large part of history of the ancient world took place, grew and had been leaving many marks behind. Many advanced ancient civilizations rose to power and the territories were allowed to grow and prosper and virtually became 'good land' between the East and the West.

Many cultures, languages, customs, traditions, religions have been modifying, transforming, changing and progressing towards several lifestyles which became part of history and have been acting as factors influencing the patterns of history and affecting it in many ways and leaving their marks to be understood and studied.

A 'Mediterranean Diet' is a diet which means more than just food and it is a way of embracing life in a way that you start finding it to be more fulfilling while showing you a path that leads towards peace of mind, happiness, contentment of soul in every day endeavor. It helps in making one more active and making life more meaningful, engaging in various purposeful and productive activities. Integration of the principles of Mediterranean Diet will need understanding of the importance of various foods and life aspects.

Initially leaving your current pattern and switching to Mediterranean can become a little daunting. Once you develop the habits of its pattern, you will find it to be beneficial in many ways. Knowledge of how to integrate a wide variety of herbs and spices, discovering ways of utilizing whole grains, beans, lentils, and legumes and adopting good and healthy ways of cooking these, all are needed for really good results.

What does the diet consist of?

The Mediterranean diet consists of a wide variety of health giving foods, herbs and spices. Each specific area of the region shows typical constituents of their dietary makeup. Many foods could be noted to have common factors that make it distinguish from the rest.

Many other factors also contribute to the intake of diet and one such factor consist of making meal times happier times for every-one. Socialization is being encouraged and meal consumption in groups is being fortified which helps in strengthening family bonds as well as social bonds. Eating in groups has many good aspect and positive sides to it.

In Egypt many foods are common part of their cuisine which include onion, garlic, tomato, olive oil, egg plants, squashes, peppers, mushrooms, cucumber, artichokes, okra, leafy green vegetables, legumes, lentils, chickpeas, fava beans, etc.

A typical French cuisine may make use of certain food items which distinguishes it from the rest and which may include white kidney beans, fresh herbs, rosemary, basil, cilantro, parsley, mint, dill, fennel, oregano, etc.

A Mediterranean diet highlights on using fish and other sea food at-least twice weekly. A wide variety of treasures from aqua are part of the meals. Many white fleshed fish e. g. sole, flounder, grouper, etc. are being liked and consumed. The diet also makes good use of many other types of fish and sea food which may include sword fish, monkfish, eel, cuttlefish, squid, octopus, etc.

Among smaller animals of land, may include lamb, goat, sheep, rabbit, fowl, etc. Feta cheese and forth dairy rich yogurt of sheep and goat are also part of this diet. As the land could not support large herds, beef is rarely and occasionally being consumed.

Importance of various foods typical to 'Mediterranean Diet'

Importance of legumes, beans, lentils, peas and pulses

A 'Mediterranean Diet' makes good use of many sources of legumes which may include pigeon pea, chick pea, mung bean, soy bean, broad beans, cow peas, lentils, peanuts, garbanzo beans, etc. These are rich in plant sources of protein and the protein content may vary from 17 to 40 %. These also contribute significantly to mineral content of the diet by providing good amount of calcium, zinc, iron, folic acid and B vitamins. Legumes are grown on around 12 to 15

% of the earth's arable surface and account for around 27 % of the world's crop production.

These are nutrient dense foods and are easy to be consumed in a wholesome manner. They are able to deliver a wide range of nutrients within relatively few calories and helps in nourishing the body while providing support to good health. They are low in fat and high in protein, anti-oxidants and fiber.

There are around 13000 varieties of peas, legumes and lentils. These could be divided into two varieties which include mature and immature. The fresh ones are the immature ones and come under immature varieties which may include the edible pod beans, shell beans, and peas. Examples of these may include snow beans, wax beans, fresh lima beans and edamame. The mature ones are harvested from their pod when they are fully developed and dried. Examples of these may include black beans, kidney beans, split peas and lentils. All these are rich sources of protein, vitamins B complex, zinc, iron, potassium, magnesium, complex carbohydrates and fiber.

Legumes helps in increasing the satiety value of foods and helps in preventing hunger consequently leading to reduced incidences of obesity and over-weight. These are good sources of soluble and in-soluble fiber and helps in regularizing the bowel movement and maintaining serum cholesterol and sugar level. These are in-expensive sources of high quality nourishment and are able to substitute meat to a great extent. As it is cholesterol free, if it is replaced for meat sources, twice or thrice weekly will help in maintaining serum cholesterol level

within normal ranges and helps in providing protection from many heart diseases.

When consumed in combination they are better able to furnish all essential amino acids provide complete protein through plant origin.

More colorful legumes are tending to be higher in anti-oxidants. A good sense of mixing and incorporating these in meals is needed which could be learnt through recipe creation and developed as well as these could be consumed in isolation to make best use of their taste and properties.

Kidney beans, lentils and soybeans come under 'beans and legumes' category of food items and are most versatile food items and provide high quality nourishment at comparatively low cost. These are low in total fat and calories while being high in over-all nourishment. These are excellent sources of high quality plant protein, complex carbohydrates, vitamins, minerals and soluble and in-soluble fiber.

The nutritional content of these foods aids in controlling several chronic diseases and reduces the risk factors associated with diabetes, coronary heart disease, osteoporosis, obesity, chronic constipation, memory loss, migraine, high blood pressure, arthritis, etc.

These are edible seeds that grow in pods and can be used to replace or substitute beef, mutton, poultry, fish and other sources of animal protein.

If these are consumed in a combination and great variety with grains, cereals and several different types of beans and legumes, can help in providing low-cost essential amino acids needed for growth, repair and maintenance of body functions.

These are cholesterol free and low in fats and carry a potential to substitute meat completely and can be used in a variety of ways. Great recipes can be created and developed to incorporate these to enhance and improve the nutritional content, texture, aroma, appeal, color and flavor of cooked meals. An eye of an enthusiast and innovative ideas are needed to make it a routine meal item.

These are easy to store and prepare and are available the whole year around. In order to prevent many chronic diseases prevalent all around the world, these needed to be part of a regular diet. These are highly nutritious and cost effective food items and due to this needs extra consideration for their good humble existence and over-all goodness which has been over-looked for quite some-time.

These are nutritionally dense, low in calories and rich in high quality plant protein. These are also good sources of B-Complex Vitamins, Iron, Manganese, Copper, Phosphorus, Potassium, Magnesium and soluble and in-soluble Fiber.

These are low in fat and sodium and are cholesterol free.

Soybeans are also rich in Omega-3 fatty acids, Molybdenum, Vitamin K, Flavonoids and Phenolic acid.

• Helps in lowering serum cholesterol level.

• Provide adequate amount of high quality plant protein.

• Helps in maintaining serum sugar level

• Works as a detoxifying agent.

• Helps in maintaining ideal body weight for height and age.

• Helps in regularizing bowel movement.

- Helps in reducing risk factors associated with coronary heart diseases and cardiovascular diseases.

- Maintains your memory.

- Helps in preventing iron deficiency anemia.

- Sort and remove stones and extra material before soaking.

- Wash three times to remove any dirt.

- Soak for 2-12 hours before cooking; add a pinch of baking powder and 1 tablespoon of lemon juice or vinegar to help detoxify it.

- Strain and wash again.

- Cook in extra water till boiling point for at-least ten minutes (do not add salt or any kind of acid).

- Simmer, cover and cook till it gets tender.

- Add herbs and spices and cook according to individual liking.

Kidney beans, lentils and soybeans and all legumes come under cost effective highly nutritious food items and the actual prices may vary from place to place and from time to time. On the average their prices may vary from 1$ per pound to 5$ per pound. Market prices may fluctuate according to production and consumption pattern of any given area. But at any given time, these are good, low cost substitutes for meat and animal sources of protein.

Importance of eating whole grains and cereals

Mediterranean Diet makes best use of a wide variety of grains in wholesome manner. It is better and advisable to consume grains in minimally processed manner. Refining and processing removes many of the essential minerals, vitamins and fiber. These grains may include barley, wheat, bulgur, faro, Millet, rice, oats, polenta, corn, quinoa, sorghum, spelt, rye, wheat berries, etc. Grain products may include breads, couscous, pastas, popcorn, etc.

Eating whole grains instead of refined grains or grain products helps in lowering the risk factors associated with many chronic diseases e. g. type 2 diabetes, heart diseases, obesity, asthma, colorectal cancer, inflammatory disease, high blood pressure, gum and tooth diseases, etc.

Whole grains are a primary necessity of every diet and at-least half should come through whole grains. Grains are rich sources of complex carbohydrates needed to furnish energy for daily tasks. It is kind of cheap source of high quality fuel. They are low in calories, but rich in vitamins, minerals and in-soluble fiber. They also contain disease fighting phytochemicals and anti-oxidants.

Importance of eating vegetables

After grain choice come vegetable choice and 'Mediterranean Diet' emphasizes on using a wide variety of vegetables in many ways. Vegetables could be consumed in raw form or cooked form. They help in providing valuable minerals, vitamins, enzymes and soluble and in-soluble fiber.

These vegetables may include zucchini, turnips, sweet potato, spinach, potatoes, shallots, pumpkin, scallions, rutabaga, radishes, peppers, peas, onions, okra, nettles, mustard green, mushrooms, lettuce, lemons, leaks, kale, fennel, eggplant, dandelion greens, cucumber, collard greens, chicory, celeriac, celery, carrots, cabbage, Brussels sprouts, broccoli, beets, arugula, artichokes, etc.

Most vegetables help in maintaining your health and protecting you from various diseases.

They are low in total calories and are cholesterol free, low in fats and rich in vitamins, minerals and soluble and in-soluble fiber. Eating raw vegetables is more beneficial than eating cooked ones, because many enzymes, vitamins and minerals get destroyed by cooking and heat therefore minimizing the cooking process is advisable.

Eating good amount of vegetables leads to reducing risk factors associated with many chronic diseases. They contain good amount of anti-oxidants and helps in boosting the immune system, protects the skin from harmful effects of sun, improves brain function and regresses aging process. For a 2000 calorie diet, you need to consume around three cups to four cups of raw vegetables daily which is equal to around one and a half to two cups of cooked vegetables.

Importance of eating Fruits

Eat plenty of fruits on a 'Mediterranean Diet' on a daily basis for good health and protection from diseases. Eating lots of fruits helps in preventing diverticulitis, heart disease, high blood pressure, certain cancers, vision loss, stroke, etc.

On a 2000 calorie diet, you may need to consume around two cups of fruits. Many research studies have led to compelling evidence to associate high intake of fruits and vegetables with reduced incidences of many chronic diseases. Fruits are low in fat, are cholesterol free and are rich in carbohydrates, vitamins and minerals.

List of many fruits needed for good health may include cherries, carob, bread fruit, berries, banana, avocado, apricot, apple, dates, dragon fruit, durian, figs, grapes, currants, raisins, grapefruit, guava, jackfruit, jujube, lime, lemon, kumquat, kiwifruit, loquat, lychee, mango, melons, nectarines, oranges, papaya, passion fruit, peach, pear, persimmon, plum, plantain, pineapple, pomegranate, quince, rhubarb, star fruit, tamarind, tangerine, tomato, etc.

Importance of eating fish and sea-food

A 'Mediterranean Diet' gives importance to fish and sea-food consumption and these are consumed at-least twice weekly. Fish is an excellent source of good quality protein, is low in total fat and is rich in omega 3 fatty acid. One to two servings of fish may help in reducing incidences of several chronic diseases e. g. asthma, cancer, cardiovascular diseases, dementia, depression, eye problems, diabetes, pre-mature birth, inflammatory conditions, etc. Fish can be consumed for good health benefits in many ways e. g. stews, fried, baked, grilled, bar-b-q, steamed, poached, smoked, etc.

Eating fish is helpful in relieving symptoms of many inflammatory conditions e. g. psoriasis, auto-immune disease, rheumatoid arthritis, etc. If taken during pregnancy, it helps in reducing the risk factors associated with pre-mature delivery of the baby. Babies, who are fed on mother's milk, have much better eye-sight. It also helps in managing diabetes, lowers risks of developing Alzheimer's disease, helps in improving blood vessel elasticity, lowers blood pressure and blood fat and increases good type cholesterol. Eating fish as well as various other sea foods has been found to be beneficial in many ways and studies have even revealed to suggest that eating more fish can reduce chances of developing heart diseases to half.

It is low in saturated fat and high in omega 3 fatty acids and therefore helps in reducing bad type cholesterol while increasing the good type. Helps in improving blood circulation and reduces risk factors associated with thrombosis. It also helps in benefiting the joints and decreases incidences of osteoarthritis. Our eyes become more bright and healthy and eyesight is protected from age-related degeneration. It contains retinol, which is a precursor of vitamin A and it helps in boosting night vision. It is an excellent source of iodine needed for optimal thyroid function. It also contains selenium which helps in synthesizing enzymes that may protect us from cancer.

Fish and shellfish are also rich in many other vitamins and minerals needed for good health and well-being. It helps in improving our lung function by giving strength to our lungs, protects from depression, help in avoiding Seasonal Affective Disorder (SAD) and post natal depression. It gives protection to skin from ultra-violet rays and conditions leading to eczema and psoriasis.

It helps in keeping the skin firm, elastic and flexible. It also provides protection from serious inflammatory bowel disease (BD) including Crohn's disease and ulcerative colitis. Our brain is around 60 % fats and most of it is omega 3 fats, therefore it is an excellent source of food for the health of our brain and to keep it at peak condition as well as to avoid many brain related diseases.

Importance of olives and olive oil

A 'Mediterranean Diet' is rich in olives and olive oil. Eating olives and incorporation of olive oil in meals helps in reducing incidences and risk factors leading towards many chronic diseases including heart disease, cancer, inflammatory diseases such as arthritis, gastric ulcers, anemia, etc.

Olives and olive oil are rich in mono un-saturated fatty acids and are helpful in metabolizing fats than getting stored in the body. Olives contain 20 % of fats. A tablespoon of olive oil may furnish around 135 calories while eating around ten medium olives may furnish around 50 calories. Olive's tree is well known to live for hundreds of years and bear fruits which are well known to enhance the quality of human life while prolonging it at the same time.

Eating olives is even better than its oil as one is able to utilize its full nutritional potential while protecting against many diseases and improving health. Uncured fruit is slightly bitter in taste, therefore could be mixed with other ingredients to balance its flavor. In raw form they are green in color, but turn black as it ripens. They needed to be added in a variety of foods and dishes in order to avail their benefits. Studies have proven record to suggest it to contain valuable amount of nourishment and substances needed for good health.

It contains anti-oxidants and anti-inflammatory nutrients and enzymes. It helps in reducing allergy related inflammation, incidence of cancer, bone loss, osteoporosis, etc. Olives are rich in copper, iron, vitamin A, E and fiber. Around 80 %-85 % of calories from olives come through its fat content. This fat is unique in its quality and around three quarter of this fat is oleic acid which is a mono-unsaturated fatty acid. It also contains small amount of essential fatty acids which is called linoleic acid. Therefore these good quality fatty acids help in reducing incidences of high blood pressure and cardio-vascular diseases.

Olives are rich source of phytonutrient which helps in keeping all the systems of our body at peak condition. Botanically speaking, olives belong to a very specific group of fruits called drupes. There are hundreds of different varieties of olive trees which all belong to same Olea europea scientific category. "Olea" is a Latin word for oil denoting and reflecting its high oil content. The oldest known living olive tree in the world is around 2000 years old.

There are many varieties of olives and all are bitter tasting fruit due to the presence of phytonutrient and therefore, may need curing to improve flavor. There are three ways of curing these which include water-curing, brine-curing and lye-curing. The history of olives began at-least 5000 years ago. The world's largest fruit crop constitutes of olives and more than 25 million acres of olive trees are planted world-wide. Spain is the greatest producer of olives, followed by Italy, Greece, Turkey, and Syria respectively.

Importance of nuts and seeds

Nuts and seeds are highly nutritious food and are packed with essential fatty acids, proteins, vitamins, minerals, complex carbohydrates and fiber. Each is different from the other in nutrition content as well as its unique flavor and all are beneficial for good health and protection from diseases. There are a wide variety of nuts which could be consumed in the raw form as a replacement for snacks. These could also be incorporated in meal to enhance flavor and to improve nutrition content in whole, chopped or powdered form.

There are a wide variety of nuts available in any given area and may include walnuts, almonds, cashew nuts, Brazil nuts, chest nuts, hazel nuts, macadamia nuts, pecans, pistachios, coconut, pine nuts, candle nuts, sweet chest nut, palm nuts, jack nuts, kola nuts, peanuts, pili nuts, soy nuts.

There are also a wide variety of seeds available having many beneficial effects on health which may include sunflower seeds, chia seeds, hemp seeds, pomegranate seeds, flax seeds, pumpkin seeds, apricot seeds, sesame seeds, cumin seeds, grape seeds, etc.

Importance of dairy and dairy products

Dairy and dairy products are consumed regularly on a 'Mediterranean Diet' in moderate quantity e. g. feta, corvo, chevre, haloumi, parmigia no-Reggiano, manchego, pecorino, ricotta, yogurt, etc. Dairy and dairy products are good sources of high quality protein, energy, vitamins and minerals.

Importance of eggs

On a 'Mediterranean Diet' eggs are being consumed especially in baked goods. Eggs are rich sources of high quality protein and could easily be consumed to replace meat. Chicken, quail, and duck eggs all are common on a traditional 'Mediterranean Diet'.

Importance of meat

Traditionally a 'Mediterranean Diet' uses more chicken than other meats. After chicken moderate amount of mutton, lamb, duck are taken. Beef is rarely and occasionally consumed.

Importance of herbs and spices

In 'Mediterranean Diet' herbs and spices are used liberally to increase aroma and flavor of foods. These herbs and spices may include thyme, tarragon, sumac, savory, sage, rosemary, pepper, parsley, oregano, mint, marjoram, lavender, garlic, fennel, cumin, cloves, chili pepper, bay leaf, basil, capers, onion, cinnamon, cardamom, dill, Italian herbs, anise, etc.

These help in reducing the salt and fat content of meals while promoting health benefits by supplying anti-oxidants. Herbs and spices help in reducing excess fat and sugar stores. Historically speaking, these have been part of alternative therapies and were used as a remedy to treat many common ailments.

Importance of drinking water

Water comes under one of the basic six nutrients needed by a human body. This nutrient has always been neglected and underestimated for its benefits. This nutrient is needed to make up for the daily losses occurring through skin evaporation, breathing and excretory system. Extra water may be needed in warm climatic conditions, during vigorous exercise and increased physical activity, at high altitudes, etc.

It helps in maintaining the fluid balance in your body. Our body is composed of 60 % of water and this water is responsible in one way or the other in maintaining the body temperature, transportation of various nutrients, production of digestive juices, circulation, digestion and absorption. Feeling of thirst is a sign that your body is in need of water and this need not be ignored. It is always better to satisfy your thirst through clean and clear water which is free from all sorts of calorie, additives and chemicals. A 'Mediterranean Diet' encourages use of more water for drinker.

Why people on the 'Mediterranean Diet' socialize at meal time?

Socialization is one of the very important aspects of a 'Mediterranean Diet' which enhances the importance of eating food leisurely with family and friends. This kind of eating pattern is beneficial for the children of the family, develops feelings of contentment among the family, people are able to consume more nutritious food and leaves positive influence on every one specially kids and young people. Developing acceptability of a wide variety of food items at young age helps in sticking with healthier choices through-out life. 'Mediterranean Diet' has been found through studies to increase alertness, energy level and contentment.

Fast food and fast life have been negatively affecting people by reducing their content level.

Slow life with more contentment has been found to be of more success. Many weight loss diets are not balanced to support healthy living and they follow an extreme regimen which could affect negatively for long term use and could leave undesirable imbalances and deficiencies and are not always risk free. While a 'Mediterranean Diet' is a well-balanced diet and helps in leaving many good effects on overall living pattern.

A 'Mediterranean Diet' pattern provides full support to the good eating habits while reducing chances of developing many chronic diseases due to its good composition of foods. It is kind of a healthy and natural lifestyle which promotes bonding between members of the family and community and encourages increasing physical activity and providing reasons for socialization. People tend to enjoy meal time in groups and gatherings which helps in developing close contact between humanity. Human to human contact helps in slowing down the pace of life while moments of life being more appreciated. It helps in developing communities which are built on solid foundations of family strength and richness of a more balanced and valuable life.

Besides socialization, these people also like to tend to live a more balanced and healthier life by increasing their physical activity; they carry out small errands and many tasks by themselves instead of relying more on machines. They prefer to walk than use a car for simple tasks, would work on lands and do cooking themselves instead of relying on fast foods.

In this part of the world, food intake is attached with many ethical, historical and cultural values and eating food is considered to be a pleasure. The main idea behind this pleasure is sharing and caring, socialization and mingling which helps in bringing serenity, joy and happiness. Through an act of social gathering, it becomes a source of pleasure and delight for everyone. In this way, thinking is blended and views exchanged.

Relatives get together and share their life experiences with each other and come to know each other's worries and problems. Good times and bad times are all being shared which makes the life more meaningful and worthy. Time spent together helps in understanding each other well and complement each other to lessen the burden and to achieve common goals, strengthening and supporting each other whenever needed.

These help in lessening each other's burden by sharing and caring and loving each other more than ever. It also helps in strengthening relationships and family ties, bringing harmony within which makes things easier for every one and plays a vital role in lessening stress and depression within groups of communities. It becomes instrumental in gaining more knowledge through experiences of other people and come to know a lot about other things which we were unable to know before.

A sample day's menu of 'Mediterranean Diet'

Breakfast Menu

Baked Eggs with Toasted Bread

Servings: 4

Preparation time: 10 minutes. _Cook time:_ 20 minutes.

Ingredients:

4 Eggs

2 Onion, 4 Tomato, 1 Green pepper (finely sliced)

½ Cup Feta cheese (grated)

¼ C Olive oil

Salt, pepper and seasonings should be according to individual taste and liking

1 Cup Fresh Coriander leaves (chopped)

4-8 Whole wheat bread slices

Directions:

1. Heat oil in a fry pan.

2. Add sliced onion, fry till half golden brown.

3. Add sliced tomatoes, green pepper, salt, pepper and seasoning and fry till tomatoes are well cooked.

4. Add eggs. Mix well with a spatula.

5. Pre-heat the oven. Take this out in a baking dish.

6. Spread evenly. Top it with grated cheese and chopped green coriander leaves.

7. Bake for five to ten minutes.

8. In the meanwhile toast all the bread slices using little oil.

9. Take out eggs from oven.

10. Serve hot with bread slices.

Lunch Menu

Roast Vegetables with Baked Fish

Servings: 4-6

Preparation time: 20 minutes. *Cook time:* 30 minutes.

Ingredients:

1-2 pound Boneless fish fillet of choice

2 Tablespoon Ginger and garlic paste

2 Table spoons Plain yogurt

1 Cup Tomato puree

4 Tablespoon Cashew powder (Take whole cashews, roast them on a skillet, grind them in coffee grinder)

2 Tablespoon Apple cider vinegar

4 Cups Mixed vegetables (cauliflower, carrots, peas, broccoli- cut them into different shapes and sizes)

¼ Cup Olive oil

2 Cups Rice (soak it in plain water for at-least 30 minutes)

Directions:

1. Wash fish thoroughly. Let it dry by keeping it over a strainer for some time.

2. Add apple cider vinegar, ginger garlic paste, yogurt, 2-4 tablespoon of olive oil, salt, pepper and all seasoning of your choice.

3. Cover it and leave it to marinate in the refrigerator for some time.

4. Take a baking tray and spread all the vegetables in it. Pour little olive oil on top, sprinkle salt pepper and seasonings of choice. Mix them lightly with the help of a spatula.

5. Pre-heat oven at moderate temperature. Roast these vegetables in the oven till lightly golden brown.

6. Take out fish in a baking dish and spread all the pieces evenly. Bake it in the oven till golden brown from top.

7. Drain out extra water from rice and put it in a cooking pan.

8. Add 3 cups of water, salt, and some olive oil.

9. Cover and cook on medium heat till done.

10. Leave it undisturbed over a warm skillet for at least 5 minutes.

11. Prepare fish sauce in a pan. Add tomato puree, cashew powder, salt, pepper and seasoning of choice and let it cook. Add water as needed.

12. Take out fish from the oven pour this sauce over the fish and serve hot with rice and roasted vegetables.

Snacks Menu

Hummus with pita bread

Servings: 4-6

Preparation time: 10 minutes.   Cook time: 0 minutes

Ingredients:

½ Cup roasted Sesame seeds

1 Cup Chickpeas (boiled and strained)

1-2 Tablespoon Lemon juice

½ Cup Olive oil

4-6 Garlic cloves

Salt

4 Pita bread

Directions:

1. Blend all the ingredients well in a blender or food processor.

2. Serve it with pita bread.

Dinner Menu

Baked Vegetables and Nut Pasta

Servings: 4

Preparation time: 10 minutes.   Cook time: 20 minutes.

Ingredients:

1 Cup Mixed nuts of choice (roast them over skillet till lightly brown)

1 Cup Corn

1 Cup Avocado (sliced)

1 Cup Fresh beans (diced)

1 Bell pepper (dices)

4 Cups Pasta of choice (boiled and strained)

1 Cup Coconut milk

1 Cup Tomato puree

Salt, pepper and seasonings (according to your choice)

4 Tablespoon Olive oil

Directions:

1. Mix all the ingredients in a baking dish and spread evenly.

2. Bake in a pre-heated oven at moderate heat for at least 20-30 minutes.

3. Serve hot.

Health benefits of eating fish on a 'Mediterranean Diet'

Fish is low in total fat and rich in high quality protein. It contains abundant amount of omega 3 fatty acids and vitamins which include D and B complex. It is also a good source of minerals needed for good health and proper functions of the body. The mineral content may include potassium, selenium, calcium, magnesium, iodine, zinc, iron, etc.

It has been recommended that intake of fish twice weekly can help in reducing factors leading towards cardio-vascular diseases. Its composition of nutrient content is such that it helps in providing protection from many heart diseases and stroke. It helps in keeping the heart and brain healthy.

Omega 3 fatty acid has a great role to play for providing many great health benefits. Our body is unable to produce omega 3 fatty acids; therefore these must be supplied through meals. All fish contain this fatty acid some more than the others. Fatty fish are good source of this and examples may include salmon, trout, sardines, herring, mackerel, oyster, tuna, trout, eel, whitebait, kipper, etc.

Omega 3 fatty acids have been found to prevent arthritis, dementia, diabetes, Alzheimer's, ADHD, depression, high blood pressure, heart attack, stroke, abnormal heart rhythm, asthma, cancer and several brain, nerve and vision problems. It helps in improving mental and physical capability and is especially helpful during pregnancy and lactation to support mother and child health and development.

Fish needed to be consumed at least twice weekly by all age group people. It helps in promoting good health, regularizes body function and protects the body from many chronic diseases. Despite many significant sources of oily fish, it need not be consumed more than twice on weekly basis. Lean fish instead, could be consumed more frequently.

Fish is also beneficial to improve sleeping pattern, enhancing memory, increasing bone density, improving the eye sight, lowering blood pressure, relieving from PMS, preventing osteoporosis and kidney diseases, etc. It also provides protection from dyslexia, obesity, psoriasis, glaucoma, dry eyes, etc.

Most importantly, it is a super-food for healthy brain function and has the ability to provide recovery properties in all sorts of brain diseases e. g. psychosis, depression, Alzheimer's, attention deficit hyperactive disorder. There have been incidences of people coming out of coma after receiving fish oil supplements. Therefore it is best for normal functioning of our brain.

Two long chain omega 3 fatty acids cannot be produced by human body. These omega 3 fatty acids include eiconapentaenoic acid (EPA) and docosahexaenoic acid (DHA) and these needed to be taken through dietary means only. Other plant sources omega 3 fatty acids may include flax seeds and walnuts, but they can only partially convert to EPA and DHA. Eating fish helps in keeping the body in peak condition while providing protection from many chronic diseases, supporting life to fullest while prolonging it.

Eating fish also helps in keeping the skin hydrated by regulating its oil production and protecting the cells from free radical damage caused by ultraviolet rays of sun. It also provides protection against wrinkles and degenerative diseases and helps in prolonging youth. Dark fleshed fish is rich in omega 3 fatty acids. Fish is also rich in anti-oxidants.

People who consume fish regularly are less likely to eat more red meat and cheeses. Fish may also contain many contaminants found in water e. g. methyl mercury, polychlorinated biphenyls, etc. Sword fish, king mackerel and tile fish are considered to be high-mercury species and therefore these fish sources needed to be avoided during pregnancy and lactation.

Farm fish, such as salmon, may also contain little mercury. Removing the skin and fat of fish may help in removing these toxicants and minimizing its exposure. Health recommendations have been made to restrict intake of farm and wild salmon. To protect the general public from contaminated fish supply strict regulations are needed to reduce industrial waste and pollutants.

There are three types of fish i. e. white fish, oily fish and shell fish. Examples of white fish may include cod, plaice, whiting, haddock, sole and hake. While examples of oily fish may include salmon, mackerel, fresh tuna, trout, sardines, herring, etc. Examples of shell fish may include crabs, mussels, oysters, lobsters, prawns, etc. Oily fish consumption twice a week helps in reducing incidences of arthritis, cancer, heart diseases and many problematic conditions and chronic diseases.

Fish can be bought as fresh, frozen, dried, canned, smoked, etc. Fresh fish is full of natural flavor and is convenient to prepare and cook. Canning process destroys the fatty acids and therefore does not contribute much to the fat content. It is better to choose low salt varieties of smoked fish. Frozen fish has the same nutritional value as fresh fish and low salt varieties needed to be chosen.

Fish is highly perishable food item and needed immediate proper storage facility. Out of 32,000 known, described and recognized species of fish, only a small number of species are used for eating purposes by humans. Some fish are even poisonous.

Different fish have different texture for example delicate texture, firm texture and medium texture. Many commonly used fish come under various flavor categories e. g. mild flavor, moderate flavor and full flavor. A low fat fish may contain 1% fat while oily fish may contain 10-25 % of fat. It is a heart friendly and heart healthy food which needed to be consumed regularly.

Due the presence of some allergens in the shell fish many people are not able to tolerate these well. The organs of many edible fish may be poisonous. Fresh fish is odorless, but it begins to smell fishy when it starts to getting deteriorated. Incorrect and improper storage facility or practice may lead to bacterial and enzymatic action resulting in release of oxidized fats and acids. The benefits of eating fish out-weight its possible risks of exposure to many contaminants.

Health benefits of herbs and spices on a 'Mediterranean Diet'

A 'Mediterranean Diet' makes good use of many kinds of herbs and spices which helps in reducing salt and fat content of meals. Other than this, they also help in improving the flavor and aroma of food. Herbs and spices are rich sources of anti-oxidants, which help in improving good health.

Many herbs and spices have peculiar known identity attached with many nationalities and each one showing likeness and fondness for some than the other. Making use of a wide variety of all types of herbs and spices can prove to be more beneficial as they all are packed and sealed with some kind of therapeutic value and goodness held within and help in contributing positively to good health and well-being.

Herbs and spices have traditionally being consumed for the treatment of many diseases and conditions. These are known to contain anti-inflammatory and anti-oxidative properties. In traditional medicine, these have been utilized for its diuretic as well as anti-hypertensive effects. Many herbs and spices contain phytochemicals which have been found to be beneficial in reducing incidences of heart diseases and cancer.

These beneficial herbs and spices may include anise, thyme, tarragon, sumac, savory, sage, saffron, rosemary, pepper, parsley, oregano, nutmeg, mint, marjoram, mace, lavender, garlic, ginger, fenugreek, fennel, dill, coriander, cumin, cloves, chives, chilies, chervil, cinnamon, cardamom small, cardamom large, capers, bay, basil, bouquet, etc.

Herbs and spices are real "functional foods" and have a long history for being used as a medicinal and therapeutic ingredient. Its history dates back to 50000 BC. These are available in wide variety and are considered to be treasures for creating culinary delights which could be individualized according to individual likes and dislikes, and tolerances and intolerances.

These are high in phytochemical and antioxidants as mentioned before. They are even higher in antioxidants than most of the fruits and vegetables therefore needed to be added in soups, entrees, casseroles, sauces, marinades, snacks, salads, pizzas, and many more.

Herbs and spices needed to be stored properly to retain their good flavor and nutritive value. Dried herbs and spices needed to be utilized within one year of its purchase. Store them in an air-tight container. Fresh herbs and spices could be stored in the refrigerator in order to retain their freshness and crispness for a longer period of time. Label these with their name and date of purchase.

Garlic

Contains antioxidants and helps in lowering serum cholesterol level, blood pressure and bad type cholesterol. Helps in raising good type cholesterol and prevents cerebral aging. It also acts as an anti-inflammatory, anti-clotting agent and boosts immunity by acting as antimicrobial.

Ginger

Ginger contains good amount of antioxidants and could be used in fresh form or dried form. It provides many health promoting benefits and historically has been recognized to possess therapeutic value and qualities. It can be consumed in fresh grated wholesome manner or paste, powdered, oil, or juice form. It belongs to the similar plant family as cardamom, galangal, turmeric, etc. It also acts like anti-emetic, anti-inflammatory and anti-microbial. It helps in boosting immunity and improves osteoarthritis of the knees.

Basil

It is rich in antioxidants and helps in decreasing inflammation. It could be used in many ways to enhance, support and improve the flavor of different foods and could be used in isolation or in combination with other herbs and spices.

Cilantro

Contains antioxidants and helps in digestion of foods, improves sleep quality, helps in lowering blood sugar level, possess anti-anxiety effects, decreases oxidative stress and provides protection from various microbial attacks.

Dill

Possess antioxidants and antimicrobial properties. It provides protection from many infections. Dill's health benefits come through two components which possess healing powers i. e. monoterpenes and flavonoids. Dill also contains substances which possess anti-carcinogenic effects. Both its leaves and seeds are utilized for seasoning. It leaves soothing effect on stomach and provides relief from insomnia.

Rosemary

It contains anti-inflammatory, antioxidant and anti-microbial agents. It helps in alleviating muscle pain, boosts immune system, improves memory, promotes hair growth and helps in the circulatory system. It has also been assumed to possess anti-carcinogenic effect and provide protection against muscular degeneration.

Oregano

It contains antioxidants and antimicrobial properties. This herb has been used in cookery and medicine for thousands of years and it possess a great number of health benefits. It has been found to be beneficial for the treatment of UTI, PMS. GI disorders, respiratory tract disorders, skin problematic conditions, dandruff, etc.

Parsley

It contains antioxidants and anti-microbial properties. It has a history of more than 2000 years. It helps in flushing out extra fluid from the body, controls blood pressure, reduces hair loss, provides relief from pain, inhibits cancerous tumors, strengthens immunity, heals the nervous system, tones the bones, etc.

Chili pepper

It contains antioxidants and helps in increasing metabolism and therefore has been found to be helpful in reducing weight. It contains capsaicin which is a flavorless, colorless and odorless compound which is responsible in bringing fiery blast of heat in the body and induces sweating.

Frequently asked questions

Q. 1. Is 'Mediterranean Diet' a well-balanced diet?

A. 1. Yes, a 'Mediterranean Diet' is a well-balanced diet.

Q. 2. Can it helps in reducing weight?

A. 2. Yes, it can help in reducing weight, but calorie intake should be less than the calorie need or calorie out-put of the body.

Q. 3. Can it be beneficial for over-all health and well-being?

Q. 3. Yes, it helps in reducing incidences of many chronic diseases while promoting good health.

Q. 4. Do I have to follow the recipes of 'Mediterranean diet'?

A. 4. No need for you to follow the recipes, you may develop and create your own recipes. You only have to give due consideration to include food items considered important on a 'Mediterranean Diet' and make frequent use of these in a wide variety so that you are able to avail all the goodness and its health giving properties.

Q. 5. How long can I use it?

A. 5. You may follow the pattern for the lifetime for its good health promoting benefits.

Q. 6. Why is this diet given importance?

A. 6. This diet is given importance due to its many aspects which promote healthy lifestyle.

Q. 7. Do I have to strictly follow the diet for its benefits?

A. 7. No need for you to follow the diet strictly. You may keep adding good food items on daily basis, weekly basis or monthly basis according to your own preference and likes. You can only start by using olive oil in the beginning instead of other oils. Then you may proceed with adding whole grains, legumes, nuts and so on.

Q. 8. Does it possess any risk factors or harmful effects?

A. 8. No, it does not possess any risk factor or harmful effects.

Q. 9. Is socialization must for this diet?

A. 9. The idea is to consume meals in the company of family and friends to promote togetherness which helps in making meal times happier times and this way of eating leaves positive marks on overall health.

Q. 10. Is increasing physical activity very important?

A. 10. Yes, increasing physical activity is very important. You do not need to go to a gym for increasing physical activity. Many activities you can increase at home level to stay physically active and fit.

6. HEALTH AND HEALING POWER OF GREEN TEA

Green tea is being liked and consumed throughout the world now but originally it was being used in China only. It has its good aroma, specific flavor and typical caffeine content for universal likeness. It is available in a variety of different packages and blends, each is different from the other. Leaves from Camellia sinensis have to undergo minimal oxidation processing to make green tea. 100 grams of green tea contain 0.01 gram of caffeine. It is being liked and consumed all around the world also due to its unique properties, therapeutic value and social benefits.

Green tea if encouraged to replace or reduce coffee intake and consumption will help in reducing the caffeine intake to 70 percent. One cup of green tea will furnish around 25-30 milligram of caffeine while on the other hand one cup of coffee will provide around 100-150 milligrams of caffeine. But this can vary according to the different types of available green tea as well as the brewing time. Green tea helps in increasing the basal metabolic rate and it helps in efficient burning of body fat. It does not possess high amount of caffeine so it can be considered to be consumed as an alternative source of stimulants. It also has been found to be helpful in reducing heart diseases.

Green tea is also being treated for a naturally decaffeinated form for healthier choices. It has been found to possess natural antibiotic properties to kill bacteria in mouth which causes bad breath. There are still so many other undiscovered benefits of it which need in depth study. Green tea has been found to be beneficial to combat dental carries, heart diseases and effective against Parkinson's disease. Caffeine in green tea and other natural substances might be a source of providing these health benefits. Therefore switching from coffee to green tea might be a good idea. To protect the flavonoids present in green tea from getting destroyed which are beneficial in improving health, water need not be heated less than boiling temperature. A few degrees less than the boiling temperature will help in retaining all the natural goodness present inside. In this way positive healing effects of green tea may be protected from getting destroying.

Caffeine intake more than 500 milligram on a daily basis may start showing various negative symptoms in your wellbeing and good health. As caffeine in green tea is much less than other sources of caffeine, it can help in boosting your overall health. It may also help in providing beneficial positive effects on body, soul and mind. One fluid eight ounce cup of caffeine in green tea may furnish around 24-40 milligram of caffeine. The same amount of regular tea may furnish around 14-61 milligrams of caffeine. Regular tea and green tea both are available in the decaffeinated form in the market.

Caffeine in green tea may vary from one cup of tea to the other due to many reasons. One reason affecting this is total length of brewing time. Other reasons may involve the brand being used as each brand result may vary from the others. Green tea also contains amino acids L-theanine which also helps in providing calming effects besides caffeine. One myth attached with green tea is that it possesses high caffeine content than coffee. In fact green tea possess even less caffeine than regular tea.

The presence of amino acids L-theonine is responsible for providing mental alertness which wrongly being associated with the presence of caffeine in it. Many people who have tried green tea find it to be delicious and helpful in improving overall health by carrying anti oxidative properties. There are a variety of brands available to choose from in a variety of beautiful packaging.

One cannot make out from a cup of green tea and its color for the amount of caffeine in green tea. Younger leaves will provide more caffeine and the terminal bud and the leaves attached to it are most valued parts. They are sweet but contain high amount of caffeine. Consuming less than 300 milligram of caffeine is recommended by health experts. When we compare the caffeine in green tea with regular tea, coffee and cola drinks we come to know that green tea is the best alternative for low caffeine substitute available. Besides it also carry many health benefits.

China is the greatest producer of green tea followed by Japan, Vietnam and Indonesia. Few of the famous Chinese varieties of green tea include long jing, qing ding, hua ding, gunpowder, kaihua, longding, huiming, bi luo chun, rain flower, white cloud, cuijian, mao feng, jasmine, da fang, wull qing, etc. Japan being second great producer of green tea also furnish a variety that may include sencha, gyokuro, hojicha, shincha, tencha, aracha, genaicha, konacha, kabusecha, fekamushicha, tamaryo kucha, matcha, kamairicha, mecha, etc.

Green tea contains a variety of nutrient and non-nutrient compounds e, g. polyphenols, phytochemicals, vitamins, enzymes, amino acids, carbohydrates, lipids, sterols, tocopherols, carotenoids and edible minerals.

7. <u>99 PLUS HEALTHY EATING AND LIVING TIPS</u>

1.   Eat balanced diet.

2.   Eat a wide variety of foods.

3.   Eat regular meals

4.   Avoid eating outside.

5.   Eat meals in the company of family and friends.

6.   Try to include more wholesome foods in your meals.

7.   Avoid trans-fats.

8.   Avoid commercially prepared foods like chips, candies, popcorn, frozen products, French fries, commercially prepared soups, sauces, dips, drinks, syrups, mixes, etc.

9. Prepare your own syrups, mixes, frozen food items, muffins, cakes, cookies, biscuits, pizza dough, bread, etc. at home level.

10. Try to use more fresh products instead of using frozen, canned or cured products.

11. Drink plenty of water and fluids between meals.

12. Try not to consume too much fluid during meals.

13. Consume your meals slowly and in a relaxed atmosphere.

14. Do not watch T.V. while eating and pay more attention to what you are eating.

15. Chew each bite thoroughly before swallowing.

16. Do not force-feed yourself.

17. Eat what you feel like eating and what is allowed for you to stay healthy.

18. Listen to many natural food cravings and your instincts for food preferences.

19.   Avoid using salt and sugar unnecessarily.

20.   Avoid using monosodium glutamate.

21.   Avoid using preserved and processed foods containing food preservatives, artificial sweeteners, colors or flavors.

22.   Wash your fruits and vegetables thoroughly before peeling.

23.   Avoid over cooking of vegetables and fruits.

24.   Store foods at appropriate temperature, at appropriate place, in appropriate containers and for appropriate period of time.

25.   Try not to buy food items in bulk if you are not sure that you will be able to consume these within due time.

26.   Make it a habit to buy fresh and eat fresh.

27.   Pay attention to all food items for their nutrient content equally e. g. fruits, vegetables, milk and milk products, meat, legumes, beans, pulses, cereals, oils and fats.

28. Add seeds and nuts into your meals regularly.

29. Avoid consuming too hot or too cold meals.

30. Adapt recipes accordingly to suit individual liking and preferences.

31. Avoid extremism in food choices.

32. It is better to under-eat than over-eat.

33. Make food choices wisely.

34. Avoid too much intake of saturated fats and saturated sugars.

35. Try to avoid adhering to patterns of any kind of extremist's diet plan.

36. Avoid the influence of marketing tactics when making food choices and purchases.

37. Eat fish regularly.

38. Eat olives and make good use of olive oil in cooking.

39. Make good use of fresh fruits and fresh vegetables in what-ever way you feel you will be able to consume these.

40. Avoid too much use of fried food items.

41. Avoid consuming too much of bar-b-q or grilled food items.

42. Avoid intake of synthetic food supplements to overcome or prevent food deficiencies diseases, but instead make good use of all food sources in good combination to avoid and overcome these.

43. Maintain your ideal body weight for your height and age by balancing your calorie intake with your calorie output.

44. Avoid intake of alcoholic beverages as much as possible.

45. Try to include food from all food groups on a daily basis.

46. Be more practical and wise with your dietary planning.

47.   Drink milk regularly.

48.   Buy meat of grass fed animals.

49.   Add herbs and spices in your meals for their natural remedial and healing powers.

50.   Make good use of natural honey for its innumerable health benefits.

51.   Avoid synthetic beverages and soft drinks and instead make good use of plain water.

52.   Avoid drinking too much of coffee.

53.   Avoid eating too much of chocolates, sweets and desserts.

54.   Use nuts and dry fruits for snacking.

55.   Avoid skipping meals.

56.   Avoid food poisoning by storing cooked foods in refrigerator or freezer.

57.   Eat fruits instead of drinking fruit juices or smoothies.

58.   Store harmful substances away from cooking and serving areas.

59. Avoid intake of animal sources of fats.

60. Consume eggs regularly.

61. Eat a wide variety of cereals and grains instead of opting just for one type.

62. Eat trimmed portions of red meat.

63. Avoid eating too much meat.

64. Remember to include green, yellow and orange vegetables in your meals.

65. Eat seasonal fruits and vegetables.

66. Try to buy organic produce.

67. Avoid the use of micro-wave oven as much as possible.

68. Properly re-heat any left-overs before eating.

69. Raw meat utensils must be washed thoroughly with soap and water before re-using.

70. Thoroughly wash your hands with soap and water after handling meat items directly.

71. Earthenware cook wares are the best choice for cooking as these do not contain any kind of metallic residue.

72. Avoid using any substandard and aged herbs, spices, nuts, dry fruits and any other food item.

73. Keep your food items covered at all times.

74. Try to avoid any kind of direct human contact with any cooked food item if not eating.

75. Make good use of wide variety of oils e.g. olive, canola, soybean, sunflower, sesame seed, almond, coconut, etc. to include a wide variety of fatty acids in your diet.

76. Make use of very mild dish washing soaps and liquids so that these do not leave any harmful residue on dishes and cook wares.

77. Avoid using plastic containers for very hot food items.

78. Store dry food items in air-tight containers.

79. Do not heat oil till smoking temperature.

80.   Eat more raw fruits and vegetables.

81.   Try to consume more wholesome food items.

82.   Try to snack on natural food items.

83.   In cold weather try to consume more hot energizing fluids and food items to keep your body energized and warm.

84.   In hot weather consume more cold fluids and food items to help your body get some relief from the outside heat.

85.   Make good use of garlic, ginger and lemon in daily cookery.

86.   Simplify your recipes and cooking procedures for more wholesome products.

87.   Protect your foods from pets and pests.

88.   Try not to mix raw food with cooked food.

89.   Store cooked foods in proper containers and cover them properly.

90. Try to grow your own produce of fresh vegetable by having a Kitchen garden.

91. Try to avoid imported food items.

92. Make your food more appealing to the eye by good use of different colored vegetables.

93. While cooking your food try to enhance and create good aroma to trigger your appetite.

94. Pay attention to develop interesting and appealing consistency of cooked food items.

95. Be creative while cooking and use your natural food balancing and combination skills to bring out the best results.

96. Before meals try to consume some whole fruits of your liking.

97. Learn to develop more culinary skills and cook better food at

home level.

98. While cooking, be very careful of cleanliness and hygiene.

99.   Use good quality water for cooking.

OTHER HEALTHY LIVING TIPS

•   In order to stay in a constant state of being free from illness and injury, we need to develop more discipline in life and live a life that will help us to stay in peak physical, mental and spiritual condition. More attention is needed towards what needed to be eaten and what avoided and how much activity is needed on a daily basis and dealing properly with over all life approaches.

•   To achieve good health and well-being, be vigilant for all sorts of unhealthy patterns which may lead us towards chronic diseases, unnecessary weight gain, accidents or incidences of catching infections. Give more time in understanding yourself better. Have good vision for your health.

•   It is our responsibility towards our-self to keep our body, soul and mind in peak condition and free from all diseases. Clarity and strength of mind comes by keeping our physical as well as emotional health in good condition. To achieve these we need to look into all aspects and reasons behind these.

• We need to look into various reasons leading us towards emotional instability and try to overcome these by addressing them at the grass root level. Balance is needed in all areas of our life for over-all health and well-being. Imbalances could lead to disaster and needed to be tackled at early stages only.

• Imbalances at any point and any sphere dealing with health may leave negative marks which could impact over-all health. Better alternatives are needed to overcome these for more beneficial health conditions. Until and unless we learn and gain vision of what good health means and stick with the right choices we may not be able to achieve balance in all areas needed.

• Experimenting on our body by applying all the available resources un-wisely could lead towards a road of disaster which may affect our health negatively. Wise decision making is crucial when dealing with matters of health to overcome the miseries and achieving success.

• Thinking in all directions while dealing with health matters can leave lasting marks on health which could either be positive or negative depending on the choices made. An insight into the depth of the matter is needed for good results. Adopting one and neglecting others will not be able to bring much fruitful results.

• Healthy living and healthy life style choices helps in making the life more easier by allowing people to live more fulfilled and contented life. They are better able to achieve more and better through their lives while making them more capable of achieving success through independent means.

• Healthy living style helps in making the best use of ones capabilities and potentials. It enhances people's self-confidence by better results achieved through healthier living pattern.

It promotes self-awareness and means of gaining good health in any given circumstances.

• One need to know and fully understand the meaning of healthy living and all the aspects and related areas it deals with. It helps in making people more productive and resilient to many difficult paths, therefore these need not be ignored if we want to achieve good results from our life.

• Due considerations needed to be given to make lifelong changes for best possible outcome in order to stay healthy and to prolong life. Eating a well-balanced diet, getting enough rest and sleep, increasing physical activity and avoiding factors leading towards more stress-full and depressive life are all important for healthy living.

• Deep understanding of the foundations and basis of good health and healthy living may be helpful in avoiding and preventing many diseases leading towards unhealthier, less productive and un-contented life. Good understanding of the factors leading towards many chronic diseases, obesity and sources of depression needed to be looked into.

• To lead a more beneficial healthy life, one need to get aware of the root causes for healthier as well as unhealthier living choices available while sticking with only the healthier ones and possible changes needed to move towards healthier living.

• Staying mentally active has been found to be beneficial and emotionally rewarding. People who love to stay mentally active have less chances of developing Alzheimer's. There is no age for learning which is a continuous process and helps in improving mental capabilities and capacities.

• Learning helps in keeping the mental health at peak condition and learning through reading is the most practical and easier way of giving an exercise to brain by people belonging to all age group. More challenging topic selection for learning will help in boosting mental capacity

• Good mental health is very important for overall good health as all our body systems are dependent on our brain function and signals sent by it. Therefore our brain has total influence on the working of all our body systems. Brain health is important for over all good health.

• Giving due attention to our brain and keeping it healthy, free from all kind of diseases will need in-depth understanding of its working. Positive thinking and optimism helps in improving brain function and its capacity. All decision making should be based on this approach and the outcome needed to be handled with positivity.

• Besides optimism, a well-balanced and nutritious diet, enhanced mental challenging conditions, and proper handling of routine stress may contribute towards, good mental capacities and capabilities.

• Sharing and caring and being respectful of individual differences helps in gaining insight leading towards more happy moments and better relationships. Socialization in its true sense helps in leaving positive marks on healthy living and all good gestures needed to be reciprocated in order to gain emotional strength and stability.

• Solving puzzles and instigating various approaches leading towards better and enhanced mental exercises are also helpful for overall good mental health. Any game or activity which engages the mind to work an extra mile helps in strengthening mental power by keeping more active, productive and well occupied.

• Keeping close to people who make you happy, enrich your life, are a source of contentment, contribute positively towards good mental health. Discuss with them your worries, fears, and thoughts. Share your good times with them and become a source of happiness for them. Try to be in the company of people you like and feel comfortable with.

• True happiness is very important for overall good mental and physical health. Keeping a close contact with friends and family is helpful in keeping one happier, contented and living a life that is more meaningful. Understand yourself better and then try to understand others better so that you find harmony towards the road of healthy living.

8. <u>*99 PLUS HEALTHY, NUTRITIOUS AND INTERESTING RECIPES*</u>

<u>*SALADS FOR GOOD HEALTH*</u>

<u>*CHEESE SALAD*</u>

<u>*INGREDIENTS*</u>

1C Cottage cheese (cubed)

½ C Peas (boiled)

½ C Corn kernels (boiled)

½ C French beans (sliced)

½ C Carrots (cubed)

1 Teaspoon Mustard Seeds

1 Tablespoon Apple cider vinegar or lemon juice

3 Tablespoon Olive oil

Salt and Black pepper (to taste)

METHOD

1.	Fry mustard seeds in oil till golden brown.

2.	Add peas, corn, French beans and carrots and fry.

3.	Add cottage cheese and fry.

4.	Add lemon juice, salt and pepper and mix well.

5.	Serve.

CHICKEN AND GARLIC SALAD

INGREDIENTS

1 lb. Chicken (boneless cubes)

1 Tablespoon Green chili paste (substitute-red chili powder or black pepper powder)

2 Tablespoon Garlic paste

¼ C Soy sauce

2 Tablespoon Lemon juice

½ C Corn flour

2 Tablespoon Honey

1 C Spring onion (sliced)

1 C Iceberg (sliced)

1 C Carrot (sliced)

1 C Potato (boiled)

Salt (to taste)

Oil (for shallow frying of chicken pieces)

METHOD

1.   Marinade boneless chicken cubes in garlic paste, chili paste, soy sauce, corn flour and little salt for some time.

2.   Shallow fry chicken pieces till golden brown.

3.   Add rest of the ingredients and move away from stove.

4. Mix well and add salt as required.

5. Serve.

MIXED VEGETABLES SALAD

INGREDIENTS

1 Cucumber (diced)

2 Tomatoes (diced)

1 C Lettuce (diced)

1 Apple (diced)

1 Cup peas (boiled)

¼C Tomato ketchup

½ C Mayonnaise

1 Tablespoon Lemon juice

2 Tablespoons Olive oil

Salt and pepper (to taste)

METHOD

1. Mix all the ingredients well in a large bowl.

2.   Serve cold.

KIDNEY BEAN SALAD

INGREDIENTS

1 C Kidney bean (boiled)

1 C Corn kernel (boiled)

1 C Tomato (diced)

1 Onion (diced)

1 Green chili (finely chopped)

½ C Fresh corianders (chopped)

1 Teaspoon Cumin seeds

3 Tablespoons Lemon juice

1 Teaspoon Chili sauce

4 Table spoons Olive oil

Salt and Pepper (for taste)

METHOD

1.   Fry cumin seeds in 1 tablespoon of olive oil.

2.   Add kidney beans and corn kernel and fry.

3.   Move away from stove.

4.   Add rest of the ingredients and mix well.

5.   Serve.

CARROTS, PASTA AND MIXED DRY FRUIT SALAD

INGREDIENTS

1 C Carrot (grated)

1C Pasta (boiled and strained)

½ C Mixed nuts (roasted on a skillet and chopped)

1 Onion (chopped)

2 Tablespoon Brown sugar

1 Tablespoon Lemon Juice

½ C Mint leave (chopped)

1 Tablespoon Any Sauce of choice

Salt and Pepper to taste

2 Tablespoons Olive oil

METHOD

1.   Fry onion in oil till soft.

2.   Remove the pan from stove and add rest of the ingredients.

3.   Mix well.

4.   Serve

ORANGE AND BROCCOLI SALAD

INGREDIENTS

1 C Orange (diced)

½ C Orange juice

1 C Broccoli (steamed)

1 C Lettuce (chopped)

1 Tablespoon Honey

1 Cup Potato (boiled and diced)

1 Tablespoon Olive oil

¼ Teaspoon Mustard powder

Salt and Pepper (to taste)

METHOD

1. Mix all the ingredients well.

2. Serve.

GRILLED BEEF SALAD

INGREDIENTS

1 C Beef steak (thin long strips)

1 Teaspoon Mustard paste

1 Tablespoon Vinegar

1 Cups Lettuce (chopped)

1 Capsicum (de-seeded and finely sliced)

1 C Tomato (finely sliced)

2 Tablespoon Olive oil

Salt and Pepper to taste

METHOD

1.	Marinade beef strips in salt, pepper and mustard paste for some time.

2.	Grill meat pieces over fry pan or grill pan.

3.	Mix all the ingredients well.

4.	Serve.

MANGO WALNUT SALAD

INGREDIENTS

1 C Mango (cubes)

1 C Walnuts (chopped)

1 Tablespoon Fresh cream

1 Tablespoon Yogurt

METHOD

1.	Mix all the ingredients well in a bowl and keep it in the refrigerator for some time.

2.	Serve cold.

CHICKPEA SALAD

INGREDIENTS

2 C Chickpeas boiled (strained)

1 C Potatoes (boiled and diced)

1 Onion (finely chopped)

1 Tomato (finely chopped)

½ C Coriander (finely chopped)

½ C Mint leaves (finely chopped)

1 Green chili (finely chopped)

¼ C Tomato paste

½ C Yogurt

2 Tablespoon Lemon juice

4 Tablespoon Honey or brown sugar or white sugar

Salt and Pepper (to taste)

METHOD

1.   In a large bowl mix all the ingredients well and taste for salt and pepper and sweet and sour.

2.   Serve cold.

HERBAL CHICKEN SALAD

INGREDIENTS

1 C Chicken (boneless cubes)

1 C Carrots (boiled cubes)

1 C Cucumber (cubes)

1 C Spring Onion (finely chopped)

1 C Peas (boiled)

1 Tomato (finely chopped)

1 Teaspoon Ginger paste

1 Teaspoon Garlic paste

1 Tablespoon Mixed Herbs (of choice e. g. parsley, basil, oregano, etc.)

 3 Tablespoon Olive oil (for frying chicken)

Salt and pepper (to taste)

METHOD

1. Marinade the chicken in ginger garlic paste, salt, pepper and herbs for some time.

2. Fry chicken till golden brown.

3. Add spring onion and mix well.

4. Add rest of the ingredients and mix well.

5. Serve.

MIXED FRUIT SALAD

INGREDIENTS

1 C Pineapple (cubes)

1 C Orange (cubes)

1 C Pears (cubes)

1 C Pomegranate

1 C Grapes

1 C Mango juice

1 C Banana (cubes)

½ C Cream cheese

Salt and Pepper (to taste)

METHOD

1.   Mix all the ingredients well.

2.   Serve Cold.

CREAMY NUTTY SALAD

INGREDIENTS

1 C Cucumber (diced)

1 C Peas (boiled)

1 C Carrots (diced and boiled)

1 C Cabbage (shredded)

1 C Potato (diced and boiled)

4 Tablespoon Lemon Juice

4 Table Spoon Mixed nut powder

4 Tablespoon Olive oil

½-1 C Mayonaise

1 C Milk

Salt and Pepper to taste

METHOD

1.   Fry mixed nut powder in oil and add milk slowly mixing vigorously.

2.   Add lemon juice, and mix well.

3.   Add mayonnaise and turn off the stove.

4.   Add rest of the ingredients and mix well.

5.   Serve cold.

ONION PASTA SALAD

INGREDIENTS

1 C Onion (finely sliced)

1 C Tomatoes (finely chopped)

1 C Coriander leaves (finely chopped)

1 Green chili (finely chopped)

½ C Olives (finely chopped)

1 C Avocado (diced)

1 C Pasta of choice (boiled and strained)

4 Tablespoon Olive oil

Salt and Pepper (to taste)

METHOD

1.   Fry onion in oil till it starts to caramelize.

2.   Add finely chopped tomatoes and fry till tomatoes get tender and become paste.

3.   Move from stove and add rest of the ingredients and mix well.

4.   Serve.

POTATO SALAD

INGREDIENTS

2 C Potatoes (boiled and diced)

1 C Tomatoes (finely chopped)

1 C Onion (finely sliced)

1 C Coriander leaves (finely chopped)

1 Green Chili (finely chopped)

1 Teaspoon Ginger paste or powder

4 Tablespoon Brown sugar or Honey

4 Tablespoon Olive oil

Salt and Pepper (to taste)

METHOD

1.   Fry onion in oil till it starts to caramelize.

2.   Add tomatoes and cook till tomatoes turn in to a paste.

3.   Add ginger paste, green and brown sugar and mix well.

4.   Remove from stove and add rest of the ingredients and mix well.

5.   Serve.

WHOLE LENTIL SALAD

INGREDIENTS

1C Whole Lentils (boiled and strained)

½ C Onion (finely chopped)

1 C Tomatoes (finely chopped)

1 C Coriander Leaves (finely chopped)

1 Teaspoon whole Cumin (roasted on skillet and crushed)

½C Coconut Milk

Salt and Pepper (to taste)

METHOD

1.   Mix all the ingredients well.

2.   Serve cold.

VEGETARIAN DELIGHT

DATES AND MANGO PANCAKES

Nutritional info: - Calories1009, Fats 46.5g, Proteins16 g, Carbohydrates138 g.

Servings: 3   Per serving: Calories336, Fats g15.5, Protein 5g, Carbohydrates 45g.

Preparation time: 5 minutes.   Cook time: 10 minutes.

Ingredients:

1 Mango (peel and cut in cubes)

¼ C Dates

½ C All-purpose flour

½ Teaspoon Vanilla essence

Water as required

2 Tablespoon Sugar

2-4 Tablespoon oil

½ Teaspoon Baking powder

Directions:

1. Mash mango and mix all the ingredients using water as required.

2. Heat oil in a frying pan. Pour this mixture and fry in two to three batches.

3. Serve hot with chocolate syrup or any syrup of choice.

SCRAMBLED TOFU

Nutritional info: - Calories279, Fats 20g, Proteins 10g, Carbohydrates 8.5g.

Servings: 1   Per serving: Calories279, Fats 20g, Protein 10g, Carbohydrates 8.5g.

Preparation time: 5 minutes.   Cook time: 10 minutes.

Ingredients:

½ C Tofu

½ C Coriander (chopped)

1 Tomato (sliced)

1 Green chili (finely sliced)

1 Onion (sliced)

1-2 Tablespoon Olive oil

Salt, pepper, herbs and spices to taste

1 Teaspoon lemon juice

Directions:

1. In a frying pan pour oil and sauté onion slices.

2. Add tomato slices and fry.

3. Add tofu and fry.

4. Add coriander, salt and pepper, lemon juice and cook till tender.

5. Serve hot with toasted bread slices.

MIXED CEREAL BOWL

Nutritional info: - Calories128, Fats 1g, Proteins 3g, Carbohydrates 24g.

Servings: 1   Per serving: Calories128, Fats 1g, Protein 3g, Carbohydrates 24g.

Preparation time: 5 minutes.   Cook time: minutes.

Ingredients:

½ C Mixed cereals

½ C Blue berries

¼ C Coconut milk

¼ C Almond milk

1 Tablespoon Mixed nuts (chopped)

Directions:

1. Mix all the ingredients well and serve.

VEGETABLE FRIED TOAST

Nutritional info: - Calories385, Fats 30g, Proteins 3g, Carbohydrates 28g.

Servings: 1   Per serving: Calories385, Fats 30g, Protein 3g, Carbohydrates 28g.

Preparation time: 10 minutes.   Cook time: 10 minutes.

Ingredients:

1 Bread slice

½ C mixed vegetables (boiled and mashed)

¼ C Bread crumbs

½ Teaspoon lemon juice

2 Tablespoon olive oil

Salt, pepper, herbs and spices to taste

1 Teaspoon mustard sauce

1 Teaspoon Tomato sauce

Directions:

1. Spread vegetable paste, tomato paste and mustard sauce over the bread slice.

2. Pour lemon juice and sprinkle salt, pepper, herbs and spices on top.

3. Cover it with bread crumbs.

4. Heat oil in a fry pan and fry it lightly till golden brown.

5. Turn around and toast on the other half of the slice.

SOUR AND SAUCY GREEN VEGETABLES

Nutritional info: - Calories 836, Fats 47g, Proteins 26g, Carbohydrates 58g.

Servings: 2　　　　Per serving: Calories 418, Fats 23.5g, Protein 13g, Carbohydrates 29g.

Preparation time: 5 minutes.   Cook time: 30 minutes.

Ingredients:

1 C Mixed green vegetables of choice (diced)

55g Mixed nuts

½ C Coconut milk

1 Tablespoon corn flour

1 Tablespoon Tomato Ketchup

1 Tablespoon Ginger/Garlic paste

1 Tablespoon Apple Cider Vinegar

1 Tablespoon Worcestershire sauce

 1 Tablespoon Olive oil

1/3 C Rice

Salt, pepper, herbs and spices (to taste)

Directions:

1. Sauté vegetables in oil and then add nuts, tomato ketchup, ginger and garlic paste, ACV, salt and Worcestershire sauce, and mix well.

2. Mix corn flour in coconut milk and add to vegetables, stir, simmer and cook for five to ten minutes.

3. Boil rice.

4. Serve hot with boiled rice

VEGETARIAN B B Q

Nutritional info: - Calories319, Fats 20g, Proteins 12.5g, Carbohydrates 33g.

Servings: 1   Per serving: Calories319,   Fats   20g,   Protein   12.5g, Carbohydrates 33g.

Preparation time: 5 minutes.   Cook time: 30 minutes.

Ingredients:

1-2 C Vegetables of choice (diced)

1 Tablespoon Ginger/Garlic paste

½ C Tofu (cubed)

1 Teaspoon oil

1 Tablespoon Soy sauce

1 Teaspoon Coconut powder

Salt, pepper, herbs and spices to taste

1 Teaspoon Lemon juice

1/3 C Rice

Directions:

1. Marinade vegetables and tofu in soy sauce, salt, pepper, ginger garlic paste, coconut powder, lemon juice and oil.

2. Arrange on skewers in a colorful manner and grill them over charcoal.

3. Boil rice.

4. Serve hot with rice.

VEGETABLE AND BEAN RICE

Nutritional info: - Calories 289, Fats 17g, Proteins 8g, Carbohydrates 33g.

Servings: 1 Per serving: Calories 289, Fats 17g, Protein 8g, Carbohydrates 33g.

Preparation time: 5 minutes. Cook time: 30 minutes.

Ingredients:

½ C beans of choice

½ C Mixed vegetables of choice (diced)

¼ C Tomato puree

1 Tablespoon Olive oil

1 small stick Cinnamon

1 Bay leaf

2 Cloves

Salt, pepper, herbs and spices to taste

1/3 C Rice

1 Teaspoon Lemon juice

Directions:

1. Pour oil in a pan and sauté vegetables with cinnamon stick, cloves, bay leaf and beans.

2. Add tomato puree, salt, pepper, herbs and spices, lemon juice, rice and a cup of hot water.

3. Mix well and cook covered for 1 minute.

4. Remove lid, mix well and simmer.

5. Cover and let it cook till it's done.

BAKED PASTA

Nutritional info: - Calories 533, Fats 22g, Proteins 11g, Carbohydrates 76g.

Servings: 2   Per serving: Calories 266, Fats 11g, Protein 5.5g, Carbohydrates 37.5g.

Preparation time: 5 minutes.   Cook time: 30 minutes.

Ingredients:

1 C Boiled spaghetti or pasta of choice (strained)

1 Onion (finely sliced)

1 Tomato (finely chopped)

½ C Mushrooms (sliced)

½ C Fresh grapefruit juice

1 Tablespoon Peanut powder

½ Teaspoon parsley

¼ Teaspoon Mustard powder

½ Teaspoon Paprika

Salt and Pepper (to taste)

1-3 Tablespoon Olive oil

Directions:

1. Sauté onion and mushroom slices in oil.

2. Add tomatoes, salt, paprika, mustard powder, parsley, nut powder and grapefruit juice and fry.

3. Add boiled spaghetti, mix well and cover.

4. Bake it for 10 minutes in pre heated oven.

5. Serve hot.

CHICKPEA AND VEGETABLE ROLLS

Nutritional info: - Calories 470, Fats 30g, Proteins 9g, Carbohydrates 50g.

Servings: 2 Per serving: Calories 235, Fats 15g, Protein 4.5g, Carbohydrates 25g.

Preparation time: 5 minutes. Cook time: 15 minutes.

Ingredients:

½ C Chickpeas (boiled and mashed)

¼ C All-purpose flour

¼ C Coriander leaves (Chopped)

½ Teaspoon Mustard seeds

2 Tablespoon Olive oil

½ Teaspoon Lemon juice

½ C Mixed vegetables of choice (diced)

2 Tablespoon Mixed nuts powder

Salt, pepper, herbs and spices (to taste)

Directions:

1. Knead mashed chickpeas with flour, coriander, mustard seeds, salt, herbs, spices and pepper.

2. Roll it using rolling pin and board, and cook it on medium hot skillet, spread a tablespoon of oil on both sides, cook on both sides till done.

3. Pour a tablespoon of oil in a frying pan and fry vegetables in it.

4. Add lemon juice and nuts powder and mix.

5. Fill your chickpea wrap with these cooked vegetables, roll it and serve.

MIXED VEGETABLE CUTLET

Nutritional info: - Calories 310, Fats 15g, Proteins 5g, Carbohydrates 31g.

Servings: 1   Per serving: Calories 310, Fats 15g, Protein 5g, Carbohydrates 31g.

Preparation time: 10 minutes.   Cook time: 30 minutes.

Ingredients:

1 Potato (boiled and mashed)

1 Carrot (boiled and mashed)

¼ C Peas (boiled and mashed)

½ C Cauliflowers (boiled and mashed)

1 Onion (finely chopped)

1 Teaspoon lemon juice

½ C bread crumbs

Salt, pepper, herbs and spices to taste

 Olive oil (for shallow frying)

½ Teaspoon Paprika

Directions:

1. Mix all the vegetables together.

2. Add salt, pepper, herbs, spices, lemon juice, paprika and mix.

3. Make a round cutlet; coat it with bread crumbs and shallow fry on both sides till golden brown.

4. Serve hot with tomato ketchup.

MIXED VEGETABLE BALLS

Nutritional info: - Calories 300, Fats 17g, Proteins 5g, Carbohydrates 35g.

Servings: 1   Per serving: Calories 300, Fats 17g, Protein 5g, Carbohydrates 35g.

Preparation time: 10 minutes.   Cook time: 10 minutes.

Ingredients:

1 Potato medium sized (boiled and mashed)

½ C mixed vegetables (boiled and mashed)

½ Teaspoon Cilantro

½ Teaspoon lemon juice

28gm Corn meal

Salt and pepper to taste

Oil for deep frying

½ Teaspoon Basil

Directions:

1. Mix salt, pepper, cilantro, basil, lemon juice in mashed potato well.

2. Make three to four small round balls of mashed potato and coat them well with corn meal.

3. Deep fry till golden brown.

4. Serve hot with ketchup.

CHOCOLATE AND DRY FRUITS CAKE

Nutritional info: - Calories 1196, Fats 117.5g, Proteins 30g, Carbohydrates 167g.

Servings: 6   Per serving: Calories 319, Fats 19.5g, Protein 5g, Carbohydrates 28g.

Preparation time: 10 minutes.   Cook time: 60 minutes.

Ingredients:

½ C All-purpose flour

½ C Mixed Dry fruits and nuts (chopped)

½ C Coconut cream

2 Tablespoon C Margarine

½ C sugar

1 Teaspoon baking powder

½ C Coconut water

½ C Chocolate chips (non-dairy)

Directions:

1. Preheat the oven at medium heat.

2. Mix all the ingredients well. Fill in muffin cups or dish and bake until done.

GREEN VEGETABLE SANDWICH

Nutritional info: - Calories 407, Fats 22.5g, Proteins 7g, Carbohydrates 32.8g.

Servings: 1   Per serving: Calories 407, Fats 22.5g, Protein 7g, Carbohydrates 32.8g.

Preparation time: 5 minutes.   Cook time: 5 minutes.

Ingredients:

2 Slices bread

½ C Coriander leaves

½ C Mint leaves

1 Green chili

1 C Cucumber (sliced)

½ C Bell pepper (diced)

¼ C Desiccated coconut

1 Teaspoon lemon juice

1 Tablespoon Margarine

1 Teaspoon mustard sauce

Salt and pepper to taste

Directions:

1. In a food processor chop all the ingredients except bread, margarine and cucumber.

2. Toast bread slices using little oil on both sides.

3. Spread margarine over bread slices.

4. Spread green spread prepared in the chopper on bread slice.

5. Top it with slices of cucumber and cover it with other half of bread slice.

MIXED VEGETABLES SANDWICH

Nutritional info: - Calories 275, Fats 15g, Proteins 6g, Carbohydrates 30g.

Servings: 1   Per serving: Calories 275, Fats 15g, Protein 6g, Carbohydrates 30g.

Preparation time: 5 minutes.   Cook time: 5 minutes.

Ingredients:

2 Slices bread

1 Tomato (sliced)

1 Cucumber (sliced)

Few leave Lettuce, mint and coriander

2 Tablespoon Mustard sauce

1 Tablespoon Tomato sauce

1 Table spoon Margarine

Salt and pepper to taste

Directions:

1. Toast bread slices using little oil.

2. Spread margarine on slices.

3. Arrange cucumber and tomato slices and lettuce, mint, and coriander leaves over bread slice.

4. Pour mustard sauce over vegetables layer.

5. Sprinkle little salt and pepper, cover with other bread slice and cut diagonally.

TOMATO AND ONION SANDWICH

Nutritional info: - Calories 340, Fats 20g, Proteins 6g, Carbohydrates 30g.

Servings: 1   Per serving: Calories 340, Fats 20g, Protein 6g, Carbohydrates 30g.

Preparation time: 5minutes.   Cook time: 5minutes.

Ingredients:

2 Bread slices

1 Onion (sliced)

1 Tomato (sliced)

Few Lettuce leaves

1 Teaspoon olive oil

1 Tablespoon Nut spread

Salt and pepper to taste

1 Teaspoon lemon juice

Directions:

1. Lightly toast bread slices using little oil.

2. Spread nut spread on slices.

3. In a teaspoon full of olive oil sauté sliced onion till caramelized or lightly discolored. Add lemon juice and mix.

4. Take one slice of bread and arrange sliced tomatoes and lettuce leaves on top.

5. Pour caramelized onion on top and sprinkle salt and pepper.

VEGETABLE AND COCONUT BUTTER SANDWICH

Nutritional info: - Calories 275, Fats 15g, Proteins 6g, Carbohydrates 33g.

Servings: 1   Per serving: Calories 275, Fats 15g, Protein 6g, Carbohydrates 33g.

Preparation time: 5 minutes.   Cook time: 5minutes.

Ingredients:

2 Slices bread

½ C Mixed vegetables (roasted and mashed)

Few Lettuce leaves

1 Tablespoon Tomato ketchup

1 Tablespoon coconut butter

Salt and pepper to taste

Directions:

1. Lightly toast bread slices from both sides using little oil.

2. Spread coconut butter on toasted slices.

3. Spread roasted and mashed vegetables on buttered slices.

4. Pour tomato ketchup on top.

5. Sprinkle little salt and pepper, cover with other slice and serve.

CHICKPEA RICE

Nutritional info: - Calories 433, Fats 15g, Proteins 12g, Carbohydrates 70g.

Servings: 1   Per serving: Calories 433, Fats 15g, Protein 12g, Carbohydrates 70g.

Preparation time: 5 minutes.   Cook time: 30 minutes.

Ingredients:

½ C White chickpeas (boiled)

1 Potato (fried)

¼ C Tomato puree

2 Tablespoon Soy sauce

1 Teaspoon Lemon juice

1/3 C Rice

1 Tablespoon oil

Salt and pepper according to individual liking

1 Onion

3 Cloves garlic

2 Pinch Mix spice powder

Directions:

1. Sauté onion and garlic till light golden brown.

2. Add chickpeas, tomato puree, lemon juice, soya sauce, mix spice powder, and salt.

3. Fry all ingredients for few minutes.

4. Add rice and one cup hot water.

5. Mix well cover and simmer.

6. When half done, add fried potatoes.

7. Cover and let it cook till done. Keep it covered over medium hot skillet for five more minutes.

SPICY ROAST VEGETABLES

Nutritional info: - Calories 483, Fats 54g, Proteins 6g, Carbohydrates 27g.

Servings: 1   Per serving: Calories 483, Fats 54g, Protein 6g, Carbohydrates 27g.

Preparation time: 5 minutes.   Cook time: 30 minutes.

Ingredients:

1/3 C Cauliflower (diced)

1/3 C Avocado (diced)

1/3 C Carrots (diced)

1 C Boiled sweet potato

½ C Coconut milk

1 Teaspoon margarine

1 Tablespoon Olive oil

1 Teaspoon paprika

Salt, pepper, herbs, spices according to individual liking and taste

Directions:

1. Pre-heat oven at medium temperature.

2. In a baking dish spread all vegetables except sweet potato.

3. Pour olive oil on top and sprinkle little salt, pepper and any herb of your choice.

4. Mix lightly and bake till light golden brown.

5. In a sauce pan bring coconut milk to boil.

6. Mix sweet potato with margarine, salt and pepper.

7. Now add coconut milk in sweet potato and beat vigorously till done.

VEGETABLE BURGER

Nutritional info: - Calories 418, Fats 15g, Proteins 12g, Carbohydrates 63g.

Servings: 1   Per serving: Calories 418, Fats 15g, Protein 12g, Carbohydrates 63g.

Preparation time: 5 minutes.   Cook time: 30 minutes.

Ingredients:

1 Bun

½ C Beans of choice (boiled and strained)

½ C Mixed vegetables of choice (boiled and strained)

1 Teaspoon lemon juice

Few leaves lettuce

1 tomato (sliced)

1 Tablespoon tomato sauce

1 Tablespoon mustard sauce

1 Tablespoon olive oil

Salt, pepper and herbs to taste

Directions:

1. Mix and mash together beans, vegetables, lemon juice, salt pepper and herbs.

2. Make a Pattie of this and fry in little oil till golden brown from both sides.

3. Toast your buns lightly from both sides using little oil.

4. Arrange Pattie, sauces and raw vegetables according to individual liking.

5. Serve with sauces of choice.

VEGAN NOODLES

Nutritional info: - Calories 468, Fats 28g, Proteins 12g, Carbohydrates 50g.

Servings: 1   Per serving: Calories 468, Fats 28g, Protein 12g, Carbohydrates 50g.

Preparation time: 5 minutes.   Cook time: 30 minutes.

Ingredients:

¼ C Tofu

¼ C Broccoli (diced)

¼ C Nuts (chopped)

1 C Noodle (boiled and strained)

3 Cloves garlic (diced)

2 Tablespoon Soy sauce

1 Tablespoon coconut oil

1 Teaspoon lemon juice

Salt and seasoning according to individual liking

Directions:

1. In a fry pan pour oil.

2. Add diced cloves and fry till golden brown.

3. Add tofu and fry.

4. Add rest of the ingredients, mix well, simmer and let it cook for five more minutes.

5. Serve hot.

ORANGE AND ALMOND DELIGHT

Nutritional info: - Calories 400, Fats 15g, Proteins 3.5g, Carbohydrates 70g.

Servings: 1   Per serving: Calories400, Fats 15g, Protein 3.5g, Carbohydrates 70g.

Preparation time: 5 minutes.   Cook time: 5 minutes.

Ingredients:

½ C Orange cubes

½ C Gelatin free jelly (set and refrigerate)

¼ C Almond milk

¼ C Figs

Directions:

1. Mix all the ingredients well.

2. Cover and refrigerate.

3. Serve cold.

MIX FRUIT DELIGHT

Nutritional info: - Calories 903, Fats 54g, Proteins 14g, Carbohydrates 135g.

Servings: 4   Per serving: Calories 226, Fats 13.5g, Protein 3.5g, Carbohydrates 33.75g.

Preparation time: 5 minutes.   Cook time: minutes.

Ingredients:

½ C Raisins

½ C Mixed nuts (chopped)

1 C castor sugar

1 C Almond milk

Directions:

1. Mix all the ingredients in a bowl.

2. Cover and refrigerate.

MANGO BALLS

Nutritional info: - Calories 540, Fats 23.5g, Proteins 8, Carbohydrates 75g.

Servings: 3   Per serving: Calories 180,
Fats 7.5g, Protein 2.5g, Carbohydrates 25g.

Preparation time: 5minutes.   Cook time: 10
minutes.

Ingredients:

1 Mango

½ C Corn flour

2 Tablespoon sugar

¼ C Almond milk

¼ Teaspoon baking powder

Oil for deep shallow frying

Directions:

1. Mash mango and mix rest of the ingredients in it.

2. Heat oil for shallow frying.

3. With the help of a tablespoon pour one tablespoon of mango paste in medium hot oil and do the same with the rest of the paste.

4. Cook till golden brown.

5. Serve hot.

VERMICELLI PUDDING

Nutritional info: - Calories 1866, Fats 114g, Proteins 40g, Carbohydrates 196g.

Servings: 6   Per serving: Calories 311, Fats 19g, Protein 7g, Carbohydrates 32g.

Preparation time: 5 minutes.   Cook time: 10 minutes.

Ingredients:

1C Vermicelli

½ C Mixed chopped nuts

½ C Sugar

1 C Almond milk

½ Teaspoon Essence of choice

1 C Water

Directions:

1. In a sauce pan bring coconut milk to boil.

2. Add all the ingredients in it.

3. Mix well, cover and simmer.

4. Cook for five minutes or till it dries up.

5. Take it out in a container, cover and refrigerate it at room temperature.

PALEO-VEGAN SMOOTHIES

A paleo or Paleolithic diet is a modern version or copied- model of what caveman in the Paleolithic era was able to consume and is commonly referred to as stone-age diet, hunter gatherer's diet and caveman's diet. It includes all plants and animal sources of foods which were habitually consumed by many hominid species during that era.

TIPS ON A PALEO DIET

• Eat and drink only when you are hungry and thirsty.

• Do not over-indulge in foods.

- Proceed gradually, one step at a time.

- Adapt recipes according to your individual taste and liking.

- Be practical and flexible in your approach.

GETTING WELL AWARE OF HIGH SUGAR FOOD SOURCES ON A PALEO DIET

In this diet, sugars in a concentrated form, is being advised to restrict. Concentrated forms of sugars may include white granulated table sugar, molasses, glucose, lactose and fructose. All carbohydrates are made up of complex starches, soluble and insoluble fibers, and a variety of sugars.

There are various types of natural sugars found in nature e. g. lactose sugar is found in milk and milk products, sucrose in cane sugar, maltose in malt, fructose in fruits, glucose in fruits and vegetables. Honey contains galactose sugar. Raw, local and un-processed honey is allowed on a paleo diet. Consuming fruits is better than juices due to its fiber content. Sugars needed to be avoided on this diet and its intake will depend on the choices you made during selection.

When we talk about avoiding sugars, we have to take into consideration the presence of sugars in all the naturally occurring sources of it. Soft dry fruits e. g. figs, dates, raisins, dried mangoes, dried apricots all contribute towards sugar and total carbohydrate overload. Your carbohydrate intake should be according to your need depending upon activity factor, body weight, condition, disease factor, etc. Plant sources of foods are rich in carbohydrates. Your carbohydrates curve ranges between various parameters starting from allowable; it leads to desirable and ends at being healthy.

Consuming more than 300 gm. on a daily basis comes in the danger zone. While consuming 150 gm. − 300 gm. means insidious weight gain. Carbohydrates intake of 100 gm.-150 gm. may help in maintaining weight. Intakes between 50 gm.-100 gm. may help in losing weight. Less than 50 gm. will help in catabolizing the adipose tissues and will help in metabolizing and burning of more fat stores. According to various diet recommendations for paleo diet, 56-65 percent of total energy should come through animal food sources and only 36-45 percent needs to come through all the plant sources of food.

FACTS ABOUT PALEOLITHIC ERA

• People usually slept to their hearts content.

• At times they survived on only one type of food for days.

• They knew how to adapt according to their resources

• They lived a minimal life.

Since last 45 years there has been a lot of controversies going on regarding what foods needed to be included and what needed to be avoided. Recently, a paleo diet has gained a more liberal and specific approach to make it better suited to a vast majority of global population.

PALEO VEGAN AND OTHER SMOOTHIE RECIPES

COCO PINE DATES SMOOTHIE

Ingredients

Coconut Milk Powder	1tbsp.
Pineapple pieces	½ C
Kiwi	1
Dates	1
Water	1C
Ice	½ C

Method

Blend all the ingredients well in a blender and enjoy.

Servings-1

Calories-162

A smoothie which is high in potassium, vitamins and fiber.

MINT PEACH DELIGHT SMOOTHIE

Ingredients

Mint leaves	12-15
Cucumber	1
Peach	1
Figs	1
Water	1C

Method

Blend all the ingredients together well.

Servings-1

Calories-125

This is a really good refreshing drink in a hot summer season.

ROSE PETAL AND CHERRIES SMOOTHIE

Ingredients

Rose Petals	¼ C

Cherries	12 large
Orange	1
Almond milk	1 C
Honey	1 tsp.
Water	1 C
Ice	½ C

Method

Blend all the ingredients well.

Servings-1

Calories- 195

This unique combination makes it a super unique smoothie with all the goodness of rose petals.

CHOCOLATE SMOOTHIES

STRAWBERRY BANANA CHOCOLATE SMOOTHIE

Ingredients

Cacao powder	½ tsp.
Banana	1
Strawberries	¾ C
Almond milk	1 C
Coconut milk powder	1 tbsp.
Water	1 C
Ice	½ C

Method

Mix all the ingredients and blend them in a blender. If it is too thick then add more water and blend.

Servings- 1

Calories- 260

This smoothie is low in calories but high in nutrition and it can be used as a supplement to replenish the needed energy after increased physical activity or exercise.

MANGO RASPBERRY CHOCOLATE SMOOTHIE

Ingredients

Cacao powder	1 tbsp.
Raspberries	1 C
Sunflower seeds	1 tbsp.
Mango	1 small
Water	1 C
Ice	½ C

Method

Blend, all the ingredient well in a blender

Servings- 1

Calories- 225

This smoothie with a king of fruits is delicious. Sunflower seeds in this can be replaced by other seeds according to individual likings and disliking. Good source of caffeine, vitamins and minerals.

BANANA AND BLUEBERRY CHOCOLATE SMOOTHIE

Ingredients

Cacao powder	½ tbsp.
Banana	1 small
Blueberries	¾ C
Olives	5
Water	1 C
Ice	½ C

Method

Blend all the ingredients well in a blender.

Servings- 1

Calories- 195

Olives are rich in good quality fatty acids. This smoothie is also a good source of potassium.

PAPAYA BLACKBERRIES CHOCOLATE SMOOTHIE

Ingredients

Cacao powder	1 tbsp.
Papaya	1 C
Blackberries	¾ C
Sesame seeds	1 tbsp.
Water	1 C
Ice	½ C

Method

Blend all the ingredients well in a blender.

Servings- 1

Calories- 225

This smoothie is heart healthy and heart friendly which is rich in fiber, and many more.

AVOCADO, PINEAPPLE AND CHOCOLATE SMOOTHIE

Ingredients

Pineapple	¾ C
Avocado	¼
Almond Milk	1 C
Coconut oil	1 tsp.
Ice	½ C

Method

Blend all the ingredients together in a blender.

Servings- 1

Calories- 195

It helps in boosting brain energy and also is a good source of vitamins, minerals and fiber.

CITRUS SMOOTHIES

ORANGE AND WALNUTS SMOOTHIE

Ingredients

Oranges	1
Dried apricots	4
Walnuts	2 tbsp.
Cantaloupe	½ C
Water	¾ C
Ice	½ C

Method

Blend all the ingredients together in a blender.

Servings- 1

Calories- 195

This smoothie is a good source of vitamins, minerals and fiber. Nuts could be replaced according to individual likes and dislikes.

GRAPEFRUIT AND CASHEW NUTS SMOOTHIE

Ingredients

Grapefruit	½
Cashew nuts	6
Raisins	2 tbsp.
Water	1 C
Ice	½ C

Method

Blend all the ingredients well together in a blender.

Servings- 1

Calories- 225

Cashew nut gives it a creamy texture and balances the strong flavor of grapefruit while raisins help in giving it a bulk.

LIME AND PEACH SMOOTHIE

Ingredients

| Lime | ½ |
| Peach | 1 |

Water melon	1 C
Olives	5
Coconut water	1 C
Honey	1 tsp.

Method

Blend all the ingredients well in a blender.

Servings- 1

Calories- 220

This one is really good and refreshing in a hot summer season. A good snack with this can make up for a whole meal.

SRAWBERRIES AND LEMON SMOOTHIE

Ingredients

Lemon juice	1Tablespoon
Strawberries	½ C
Papaya	½ C
Almond milk	1 C

Cauliflower	¼ C
Water	1 C
Ice	½ C

Method

Blend all the ingredients together in a blender.

Servings- 1

Calories- 170

Papaya is very good for digestion and also helps in relieving constipation naturally. It needs to be a part of a routine meal planning.

BLACKBERRIES AND ORANGE SMOOTHIE

Ingredients

Mandarin orange	¾ C
Blackberries	¾ C
Macademia seeds	1 tbsp.
Coconut cream powder	1 tsp.

Water	1 C
Ice	½

Method

Blend all the ingredients well in a blender.

Servings- 1

Calories- 210

This smoothie is a good source of fiber, vitamins, minerals and electrolytes. Combination can vary according to individual taste and liking.

FRUITY SMOOTHIES

POMEGRANET AND MANGO SMOOTHIE

Ingredients

Pomegranate	½
Mango	1 small
Blue berries	¾ C

Seeds of your choice	1 tbsp.
Water	1 C
Ice	½

Method

Blend all the ingredients well in a blender.

Servings- 1

Calories- 270

For thousands of years pomegranate has been used as an ingredient of natural medicines and therapies. It has many natural healing powers which needs better understanding through studies.

APPLE AND PEACH SMOOTHIE

Ingredients

Apple	1
Peach	1
Honey dew melon	1 C

Pecans	2
Avocado oil	1 tsp.
Water	1 C
Ice	½

Method

Blend all the ingredients together in a blender.

Servings- 1

Calories- 270

It is a good source of pectin which is a soluble fiber and helps in excreting cholesterol from the body by binding with it during digestion and excreting it.

PINEAPPLE AND GRAPES SMOOTHIE

Ingredients

Grapes	15
Nectarines	1
Pineapple	½ C

Pistachio	1 tbsp.
Sesame seed oil	1 tsp.
Water	1 C

Method

Blend all the ingredients well in a blender.

Serving- 1

Calories- 270

PLUM AND STRAWBERRIES SMOOTHIE

Ingredients

Plums	2
Strawberries	1 C
Banana	1 small
Coconut milk	1 C
Avocado oil	1 tsp.
Water	1 C
Ice	½ C

Method

Blend all the ingredients well in a blender.

Servings- 1

Calories- 285

It is in a combination of majority's liking. Mostly people like to have strawberries in combination with bananas. It is rich in potassium and vitamin C.

KIWI AND RASPBERRIES SMOOTHIE

Ingredients

Kiwi	1
Raspberry	1 C
Figs	2
Raw mango	½
Almond milk	1 C
Ice	½ C

Method

Blend all the ingredients well in a blender.

Serving- 1

Calories- 240

Raw mangoes give it a little sour flavor which helps in its ingestion and digestion. Variation could be used for individual liking.

GREEN SMOOTHIES

SPINACH AND BANANA SMOOTHIE

Ingredients

Spinach	½ C
Banana	1 small
Avocado	1/8
Cashew nuts	6
Honey	1 tsp.
Water	1 C

Ice	½ C

Method

Blend all the ingredients well in a blender.

Servings- 1

Calories- 182

Spinach which is highly beneficial for good health and well-being is most of the time being avoided due to various reasons. Consuming it through smoothies makes it more practical and easier to use on a daily basis.

ICEBERG AND PAPAYA SMOOTHIE

Ingredients

Iceberg	½ C
Papaya	1 C
Dried apricots	4
Olives	5
Coconut milk	1 C

Ice   ½ C

Method

Blend all the ingredients well in a blender.

Servings- 1

Calories- 234

Olives and coconut milk makes it a good source of medium chain triglycerides and heart friendly oil.

MINT AND PINEAPPLE SMOOTHIE

Ingredients

Mint leaves	½ C
Pineapple	1 C
Cauliflower	½ C
Lemon	½
Olives	5
Water	1 C
Ice	½

Method

Blend all the ingredients well in a blender.

 Servings- 1

Calories- 129

It contains mint leaves which for century's people have been utilizing for the purpose of diet therapy to treat different diseases.

BROCCOLI AND PEACH SMOOTHIE

Ingredients

Broccoli	½ C
Peach	1
Carrot	1 small
Almond milk	1 C
Macademia seeds	1 tbsp.
Cinnamon powder	1 pinch
Ice	½ C

Method

Blend all the ingredients in a blender.

Serving- 1

Calories- 134

It is a rich source of vitamins and is low in proteins. Foods consumed in great variety in a meal helps in better absorption of nutrients during digestion.

CUCUMBER AND APPLE SMOOTHIE

Ingredients

Cucumber	1
Apple	1
Cherry tomatoes	½ C
Bell pepper	1/2
Figs	2
Almond milk	1 C
Mace powder	1 pinch

Method

Blend all the ingredients well in a blender.

Servings- 1

Calories- 202

This smoothie is a soothing drink for a hot summer afternoon due to all its natural cooling properties.

CREAMY SMOOTHIES

AVOCADO AND CARROT SMOOTHIE

Ingredient

Avocado	¼
Carrots	1 small
Lemon	½
Pine nuts	1 tbsp.
Tangerine	1
Water	1 C

Ice   ½ C

Method

Blend all the ingredients well in a blender.

Serving- 1

 Calories- 207

This smoothie is a good source of carotenoid and vitamin C. It is also rich in fiber content.

LYCHEE AND COCONUT CREAM SMOOTHIE

Ingredients

Coconut cream   1 C

Lychee's   10

Hazelnut   2 tbsp.

Mango   1 small

Green tea cold   1 C

Ice   ½ C

Method

Blend all the ingredients well in a blender.

Servings- 1

Calories- 285

This smoothie is a good source of anti-oxidant and mono-unsaturated fatty acids.

SWEET POTATO AND CHERRY TOMATO SMOOTHIE

Ingredients

Sweet potato	½ C
Tangerine	1
Cherry tomatoes	½ C
Honey	1 tsp.
Coconut oil	1 tsp.
Water	1 C
Ice	½ C

Method

Blend all the ingredients together in a blender.

Servings- 1

Calories- 222

This smoothie helps in boosting your immune system by providing protection against infection as coconut and its oil provide natural anti-biotic properties.

BANANA AND BLUEBERRIES SMOOTHIE

Ingredients

Banana	1 small
Blueberries	¾ C
Almond milk	1 C
Instant coffee	½ tsp.
Ice	½ C
Water	1 C

Method

Blend all the ingredients well in a blender.

Servings- 1

Calories- 165

This smoothie supplies good source of potassium besides other nourishment and could help in getting rid of potassium deficiency.

PAPAYA AND CHERRIES SMOOTHIE

Ingredients

Papaya	1 C
Cherries	½ C
Lemon	½
Olives	5
Almond powder	2 tbsp.
Water	1 C
Ice	½ C

Method

Blend all the ingredients well in a blender.

Servings- 1

Calories- 180

Papaya, cherries and olives make a great supplement to gain strength and provide bulk to a diet.

MANGO COCONUT SMOOTIE

INGREDIENTS:

Yogurt-   100gms.

Mango cubes-   1/2Cup

Lemon Juice-   1tsp.

Coconut milk powder- 1 tbsp.

Frozen Sugar Syrup-   4tbsp. (1cup sugar+1cup water

                            cook it for few minutes and then

freeze at room temp.)

Method

1-Add all the ingredients in a nutribullet, blend well, pour in a serving glass and enjoy.

Servings: 1

A good source of nourishment and furnishes around 200-300 calories. It is also a good source of protein, fiber , vitamin c, and medium chain triglycerides.

PEACH AND CANTALOUPE SMOOTHIE

Ingredients

Peach	1
Cantaloupe	½ C
Lime	1
Raisins	2 tbsp.
Cashew nuts powder	2 tbsp.
Water	1 C

Ice   ½ C

Method

Blend all the ingredient in a blender.

Serving- 1

Calories- 240

KIWI, BANANA AND STRAWBERRY SMOOTHIES

Ingredients

Banana   1 small

Strawberries   ½ C

Kiwi   1

Almond milk   1 C

Figs   2

Ice   ½ C

Method

Blend all the ingredients well in a blender.

Servings- 1

Calories- 265

POMEGRANATE AND PINEAPPLE SMOOTHIE

Ingredients

Pomegranate	½
Pineapples	¾ cup
Pear	1
Walnuts	2
Dried apricots	2
Water	1 C
Ice	½ C

Method

Blend all the ingredients in a blender

Servings-1

Calories-255

APPLE, ORANGE AND PAPAYA SMOOTHIE

Ingredients

Apples	1
Papaya	½ C
Orange	1
Honey	1 tsp.
Olive oil	1 tsp.
Water	1 C
Ice	½ C

Method

Blend all the ingredients in a blender.

Servings- 1

Calories- 215

PLUMS, GRAPES AND MANGO SMOOTHIE

Ingredients

Grapes	15
Plums	2
Mango	1 small
Avocado oil	1 tsp.
Almond Milk	1 C
Ice	½ C

Method

Blend all the ingredients in a blender.

Servings- 1

Calories- 270

THAI CUISINE

The national cuisine of Thailand is known as 'Thai Cuisine'. The use of strong aromatic herbs and spices is the distinguishing component of Thai food. Herbs and spices and aromatic flavor components are used in detail, balanced and variety. Four fundamental taste senses of sour, salty, sweet and bitter are used in balanced.

Few dishes are quite simple to prepare while other require creation of harmonious finished product which needs expertise. 'Thai Cuisine' is basically divided into four regional cuisines i. e. Northern, Southern, Central and Northeastern. 'Thai cuisine' has been influencing the cuisine of the neighboring countries as well as getting influenced by them.

In addition to local and neighboring influence, it is also influenced by its historical Royal Thai Cuisine. Western influence has been playing its part in modifying techniques and practices used recently. Use of coconut milk and fresh turmeric is common in Southern region, while use of lime juice is common in Northern dishes.

From 1960s and onwards, the presence of international troops led to its international recognition. According to one survey, 'Thai Cuisine' ranks at number four for its liking at international level.

Pad Thai

Ingredients:

8oz. Thai rice noodles or any noodles (boil and keep aside)

1 ½ C - 2 C Chicken boneless (cut in cubes and marinate in 1 Tablespoon corn starch and 3 Tablespoons soy sauce)

6 Garlic cloves (sliced)

2 C Bean sprouts

3-4 Green onion (sliced)

½ C Mixed nuts (chopped)

3-4 Tablespoon oil

½ C Pad Thai sauce (1/4 C tamarind paste or lemon juice, 2 Tablespoon fish sauce or mushroom sauce or Worcestershire sauce, 3 Teaspoon chili sauce or substitute, ½ Teaspoon chili powder, 3 Tablespoon brown sugar or honey or white sugar, ¼ Teaspoon white pepper powder. Mix all the ingredients well and keep aside.

Method (Serves 2-3):

1. In a fry pan add 3-4 tablespoons of oil. Fry garlic slices till golden brown.

2. Add marinated chicken cubes and fry for few minutes. Add little water, cover and simmer. Cook for five to ten minutes.

3. Uncover, add chopped nuts and mix well.

4. Add noodles, bean sprouts, green onion, pad Thai sauce, salt and mix well.

5. Fry for few minutes.

6. Serve hot.

Thai garlic prawns

Ingredients:

15 Prawns (shelled)

2 Tablespoon Soy sauce

2 Tablespoon Oyster sauce

1 Tablespoon Fish sauce (substitute-Worcestershire sauce or mushroom sauce)

1 Tablespoon Lemon juice

2 Tablespoon Garlic (minced)

¼- ½ Teaspoon Chili powder (substitute-1 fresh crushed chili)

1-2 Tablespoon Brown sugar, white sugar or honey

Oil for frying

Method (Serves 2-3):

1. Combine all the ingredients well except oil. Keep in the refrigerator for marinating for some time.

2. Heat oil for deep frying and add prawns in batches of five. Fry for few minutes and be careful not to overcook.

3. Serve hot with rice

Thai lemon grass chicken

Ingredients:

4 Quarters Chicken (with skin)

10 cloves Garlic (crushed)

½ C Yogurt or carnation milk (plain)

2-3 stalks Lemon grass

1 Onion (purple, medium)

2 Tablespoon Soy sauce

1-2 Fresh chilies (substitute- chili flake, according to taste)

½ C Coconut milk

2-3 Tablespoon Fish sauce (substitute- mushroom sauce or Worcestershire sauce)

Method (Serves 4):

1. Blend all the ingredients well in a blender.

2. Marinate washed and dried chicken in this blended marinade. Keep covered in the refrigerator for some time.

3. Take out chicken from the refrigerator and spread its content in a baking dish evenly.

4. Pre-heat oven at medium temperature and cook it in the oven till it turns golden brown from top.

5. Serve hot with rice and favorite sauces.

Thai heavenly pineapple chicken fried rice

Ingredients:

1C Pineapple (cubes)

3-4C Cooked Rice (little under-cooked)

1C Chicken (boneless cubes)

6 cloves Garlic (sliced)

1C Cashew nuts (Whole and lightly roasted)

½ C Spring Onion (sliced)

1C Peas

4 Tablespoon Oil

4 Tablespoon Soya Sauce

Method (Serves 3-4):

1. Fry garlic slices in oil till golden brown.

2. Add chicken and cook till tender at low heat.

3. Add cashew nuts, peas, spring onion, and fry for some time.

4. Add rice and drizzle soya sauce over it. Mix well and fry on medium heat for few minutes.

5. Add pineapple cubes, mix and fry for one more minute.

6. Serve hot.

Thai chicken curry

Ingredients:

1 lb. Chicken (boneless cubes)

2 Potatoes (peel and cut in quarters)

2 Tomatoes (chopped)

1 Onion large (sliced)

1 C Coconut milk

2 Tablespoon Ginger garlic paste

1 Teaspoon Turmeric powder

1 Teaspoon cumin seeds

½C Oil

Salt and extra seasonings and sauces (according to individual taste and liking)

Method (Serves 3-4):

1. Fry onion in oil till light golden brown.

2. Add rest of the ingredients except coconut milk.

3. Fry for some time till tomatoes become paste and chicken develops flavor.

4. Add coconut milk and bring to boil.

5. Simmer, cover and let it cook till chicken and potatoes get tender.

6. Add salt, seasonings and sauces according to your liking. Add little water and cook to acquire required consistency at low heat.

7. Serve hot with rice.

Thai Chicken sate

Ingredients:

1 lb. Chicken (boneless cubes)

¼ C Coconut cream

1 Shallot (finely sliced)

2 Tablespoon Ginger garlic paste

2 Tablespoon Soy sauce

1 Tablespoon Brown sugar

1 Tablespoon Lemon juice

Salt (according to taste)

Method (Serves 3):

1. Mix all the ingredients well in a bowl, cover and keep it in the refrigerator for some time for marinating.

2. Use pre-soaked bamboo skewers for pan grilling of marinated chicken.

3. Spray little oil over a grill pan and grill these chicken skewers over medium flame till medium golden brown from all sides.

4. Serve hot with favorite dipping.

Thai cashew chicken

Ingredients:

1 lb. Chicken (boneless cubes marinated in 2 tablespoon tapioca flour, 1 tablespoon rice vinegar)

1 Teaspoon Chili powder

½ C Sesame seed oil

1 C Onion (diced)

1 C Red bell pepper (diced)

1 C Water chestnut (diced)

1C Cashew nuts (lightly roasted on a skillet)

3 Spring Onion (sliced)

For Sauce

3 Tablespoon Sesame seed oil

Salt to taste

¼ C Soy sauce

2 Tablespoon Brown sugar

½C Tomato ketchup

2 Tablespoon white vinegar

Method (Serves 4-5):

1. Fry chicken in oil till lightly golden brown.

2. Add chili powder and all the vegetables. Mix well and cook on high flame for few minutes.

3. Mix all the ingredients of sauce and cook. Add little water to achieve required consistency.

4. Add this sauce to vegetables and chickens and cook together for few minutes.

5. Serve hot with rice.

Thai chicken green curry

Ingredients:

1 C Coconut milk

3 Tablespoon oil

8 cloves Garlic (sliced)

2-3 Tablespoon Green curry paste (prepare at home by blending coriander leaves, cumin seeds and green chilies together)

4 Tablespoon Fish sauce (or Worcestershire sauce or mushroom sauce)

1 Tablespoon Brown sugar

Basil leaves (according to taste)

1 C Chicken broth

Salt to taste

Method (Serves 3-4)

1. Fry garlic slices in oil till lightly golden brown.

2. Add chicken and fry for few minutes.

3. Add green curry paste, fish sauce, brown sugar, chopped chilies and salt.

4. Fry for few more minutes.

5. Now add coconut milk and chicken broth.

6. Cover, simmer and let it cook for five to ten minutes.

7. Add basil leaves and serve hot with rice.

Thai shrimp coconut curry

Ingredients:

12-15 Shrimps (shelled)

1 C Pineapple (cubes)

1C Cherry Tomatoes

1C Coconut milk

2 Fresh red chilies (minced)

½ C Onion (minced)

6 Cloves garlic (minced)

1 inch square cube Ginger (minced)

2 Tablespoon Fish sauce (substitute-Worcestershire sauce or mushroom sauce)

½ Teaspoon turmeric powder

½ Teaspoon Coriander powder

1 Tablespoon Brown sugar or white sugar or honey

1 Tablespoon Tomato ketchup

1 Tablespoon Lemon juice

4 Tablespoon Oil

Salt (to taste)

Method (Serves 3-4):

1. Fry minced onion, minced fresh red chilies, minced garlic and minced ginger.

2. Add turmeric powder, coriander powder, salt, lemon juice, fish sauce, tomato ketchup, brown sugar and fry for few minutes.

3. Add shrimps and fry for few minutes.

4. Add coconut milk, cover and bring to boil and then simmer and cook till done.

5. Add pineapple cubes and cherry tomatoes and cook for few more minutes.

6. Serve hot with rice

Thai baked fish

Ingredients:

1 lb. white fish fillet

2 Tablespoon Apple cider vinegar

2 Tablespoon Brown sugar

2 Tablespoon Soy sauce

½ Teaspoon Red chili powder

2 Tablespoon Ginger and garlic paste

2 Tablespoon Oil

1 Stalk Lemon grass (finely sliced)

2 Tablespoon Corn flour

Salt (to taste)

Method (Serves 3-4):

1. Mix all the ingredients well except fish.

2. Wash fish and dry it with a paper towel.

3. Marinade fish in the well mixed ingredients and store it in the refrigerator for some time.

4. Pre-heat oven at medium temperature and bake fish till done.

5. Garnish with fresh coriander leaves.

6. Serve hot with rice.

Thai lamb curry

Ingredients:

1 lb. Lamb (cut in small pieces)

1 Teaspoon Red chili powder

2 Tablespoon Ginger and garlic paste

1 Teaspoon coriander powder

2 Tablespoon Fish sauce (substitute-Worcestershire sauce or mushroom sauce)

1 Cup Coconut milk

½ C Basil leaves (chopped)

1 Tablespoon Brown sugar or white sugar or honey

1 Red bell pepper (sliced)

3 Tablespoon Oil

Salt (to taste)

Method (Serves 3-4):

1. Fry ginger and garlic paste in oil for few minutes.

2. Add washed and well strained lamb pieces and fry for few more minutes.

3. Add rest of the ingredients except bell pepper and basil leaves.

4. Cover, simmer and cook till meat gets tender.

5. Add little water to acquire required consistency and add bell pepper and bring to boil.

6. Simmer and cook for few more minutes.

7. Add basil leaves and serve hot with rice.

Thai chicken ginger

Ingredients:

1 lb. Chicken (boneless cubes)

6 cloves Garlic (sliced)

1 Tablespoon Fish sauce (substitute-Worcestershire sauce or mushroom sauce)

1 C Mushroom (sliced)

1 Tablespoon Brown sugar or white sugar or honey

1/2 C ginger (cut in julienne)

5 Green Onion (sliced)

1 Green chili (finely sliced)

½ Teaspoon Red chili powder

¼C Oil

Salt and pepper to taste

Fresh coriander leaves for garnishing

Method (Serves 3-4):

1. Fry garlic slices in oil till lightly golden brown.

2. Add chicken cubes and fry, add little water, cover and simmer for few minutes till chicken gets tender.

3. Add rest of the ingredients and keep frying at medium heat.

4. Garnish with freshly chopped coriander leaves.

5. Serve hot with rice.

Thai beef curry

Ingredients:

1 lb. Beef (boneless cubes)

4 Tomatoes (diced)

1 Red bell pepper

2 Bay leaves

½ C Basil leaves (chopped)

¼ C Tomato paste

1 Onion (chopped)

2 Tablespoon Ginger and garlic paste

2 Tablespoon Soy sauce

2 Tablespoon Fish sauce (substitute-Worcestershire sauce or mushroom sauce)

1 C Coconut milk

1 Teaspoon Red chili powder

½ Teaspoon Turmeric powder

½ Teaspoon Coriander seed powder

½ Teaspoon Cumin seed powder

½C Oil

Salt (to taste)

Method (Serves 3-4):

1. Fry onion and ginger and garlic paste for few minutes.

2. Add beef and fry for few more minute.

3. Add rest of the ingredients except bell pepper, tomatoes and basil leaves.

4. Cover, simmer and cook till tender. You can use pressure cooker to lessen cooking time.

5. Add little water if needed to acquire required consistency and bring to boil.

6. Add tomatoes and bell pepper and cook for few minutes.

7. Garnish with freshly chopped basil leaves and serve hot with rice.

Thai chicken cakes

Ingredients:

1 lb. Chicken (boneless)

3 Onions

3 Fresh green or red chilies

1 C Fresh Coriander leaves

8 Cloves garlic

1 inch square piece of Ginger

Salt and pepper (to taste)

Herbs and spices (to taste)

Oil for frying

Method (Serves 3-4):

1. Except oil chop all the ingredients well in a chopper or food processor.

2. Make a round flat disc and shallow fry till golden brown from both sides.

3. Garnish with lemon wedges, salad leaves, tomato slices and cucumber slices.

4. Serve hot with rice.

Thai beef noodles

Ingredients:

1 Packet noodles (boiled and strained)

1 lb. Beef (boneless, thinly sliced, boiled)

8 Cloves Garlic (sliced)

1 C Broccoli (cut into small pieces)

1 Cup peas

1 C Spring onion (sliced)

2 Tablespoon Sesame seeds (lightly roasted over skillet)

2 Tablespoon Honey or Brown sugar or White sugar

¼ C Soy sauce

4 Tablespoon Oil

Salt, herbs and spices (according to taste e.g. red chili powder, cilantro, cumin seed powder, dry basil, black pepper, etc.)

Method (Serves 3-4):

1. Fry garlic slices till golden brown and add beef and fry.

2. Add soy sauce, honey and sesame seeds and fry.

3. Add broccoli, peas, spring onion, salt, spices and herbs of your choice and fry.

4. Serve hot with boiled noodles.

FEW OTHER INTERESTING RECIPES

Beef Fried Kebabs

These kebabs are easy to prepare and store and are high in calories and protein and can be frozen for future use.

Servings: 3-4

Preparation time: 10 minutes

cooking time: 20 minutes

Ingredients:

1lb. Beef, veal, mutton, fish or chicken (boneless)

2-3 Onion

1 C Coriander leaves

3-4 Green chilies

½ C Fresh mint leaves

3 Tablespoon Ginger garlic paste (or 1 inch piece ginger and ten cloves garlic)

2 Tablespoon Lemon juice

½ Teaspoon Mustard powder

1 Tablespoon whole Cumin seeds

1 Tablespoon whole Coriander seeds

Salt to taste

Oil for frying

Instructions:

1.   Except oil, chop all the ingredients together in a chopper or food processor.

2.   Take a little chopped matter and flatten between your palms to make a round disc of around 2 inch to 3 inch in diameter and ¼ to ½ inch thick.

3.   Shallow fry these kebabs from both sides till golden brown.

4.   Serve hot with rice, sauces and salad of your choice.

Chicken Karahi

Karahi gosht (gosht means meat) is usually cooked and served in a karahi (round based pan with handles on both sides). This dish is very easy to cook and is rich in flavor, aroma and appeal. It should be consumed occasionally due to its high caloric value. It tastes best when eaten with a freshly baked nan or freshly cooked onion or garlic rice. A little variation in ingredients and cooking procedure to adapt individual likes and dislikes and tolerances and intolerances is recommended for overall benefit for individual use. It is a Pakistani dish which usually is eaten on special occasions.

Servings: 3-4

Preparation time: 10 minutes cooking time: 20 minutes

Ingredients:

1 C Onion (finely sliced)

3 Tablespoon Ginger garlic paste

1 lb. Chicken (small pieces)

3 C Tomatoes (chopped)

6-8 Green chilies (cut each into two or three pieces)

1 C Fresh coriander leaves (chopped)

1 Teaspoon Turmeric powder

1 Teaspoon Garam masala powder (hot spice powder or five spice powder or all spice powder)

1C Oil

Salt according to taste

Instructions:

1.   Heat oil and fry onion slices till light golden brown.

2.   Add ginger and garlic paste and mix.

3.   Wash chicken and drain out extra water.

4.   Add chicken and fry for five minutes.

5.   Add chopped tomatoes, green chilies, coriander leaves, salt and all the spices.

6.   Simmer and let it cook for ten to fifteen more minutes.

7.   Serve hot with rice, bread slices, chapatti, pita bread or nan and

enjoy.

Khawsuey

This dish was originated from Burma and is also known as Burmese dish. It is being liked and consumed in various neighboring countries and recipes have been adapted to suit the general population of these people.

Servings: 4

Preparation time: 15 minute   Cook time: 15-30 minutes.

Ingredients:

1 packet Spaghetti (boiled, strained)

Fresh coriander leaves, lemon slices and mint leaves for garnishing

'For meat gravy'

1 lb. Beef, chicken or veal (boneless, cut in small cubes)

2C Onion (finely sliced)

4 Tablespoons Desiccated coconut or 1 C Coconut milk

4 Tablespoons Ginger and garlic paste

1Teaspoon each turmeric powder, cumin seeds powder, coriander seeds powder, red chili powder, garam masala powder, salt

3 Tablespoon lemon juice

½C Oil

'For coconut milk curry'

1 C Coconut milk

1 C Yogurt

¼ C Gram powder

½ Teaspoon Turmeric powder

1 Onion (finely sliced)

1 Egg

¼C Oil

Salt to taste

Instructions:

1.   Prepare meat gravy and fry onion in oil till golden brown.

2.   Add ginger garlic paste, coconut powder, all spices and meat and fry for few minutes.

3. Add little water to make the meat tender, simmer, cover and let it cook till meat gets tender.

4. In a separate pan prepare coconut curry and fry sliced onion till golden brown.

5. Blend rest of the ingredients in a blender and add little water to make it little thin.

6. Add this blended mixture into fried onion and increase the flame. Keep stirring as it starts to thicken.

7. Simmer, cover and cook for five to ten minutes.

8. Spread boiled spaghetti evenly in a serving dish. Warm it up in the micro-wave oven.

9. Add coconut curry on top of spaghetti.

10. Add meat gravy on top of coconut curry.

11. Garnish with freshly chopped coriander leaves.

12. Serve hot.

9. DIET THERAPY FOR MANY COMMON AILMENTS AND DISEASES

⍰ DIABETES

There are three types of diabetes i. e. type 1, type 2 and type 3 or gestational diabetes. In type 1 diabetes mellitus formerly known as insulin dependent diabetes mellitus or juvenile onset diabetes mellitus, the pancreas are totally unable to produce insulin and therefore need insulin injections at interval are needed throughout life for survival. In this insulin injections, diet and exercise play a vital role in controlling blood sugar level. In type 2 diabetes mellitus, a patient's pancreas are able to produce insulin needed mostly but the body cells are resistant to it and therefore are unable to utilize it. Oral hypoglycemic drugs, diet regimen and exercise helps in this to control blood sugar and keep it within normal range. Around 20 % of pregnancy cases show signs of gestational or pregnancy onset diabetes. Most of these can be controlled through low carbohydrate diet and exercise but few still need to take hypoglycemic drugs along with diet and exercise. Recipes can be developed keeping in mind their diet restrictions.

In uncontrolled or type I diabetes, insulin is required therefore diet restriction is not required all the time. But in type II or controlled diabetes diet plays a major role to control blood sugar and keep it within normal range. These people need to limit their intake of carbohydrates. Cereals, vegetables and fruits are the main sources of carbohydrates. Few of these food items contain high amount of carbohydrates for example potatoes, sweet potatoes, rice, bananas, mangoes and so on. Concentrated sources of carbohydrates like simple sugar is usually fully omitted and replaced by alternatives or artificial sweetners. Rest of the food items are restricted to certain extent keeping in mind individual needs and requirements. Patients are advised to exercise to bring their extra blood sugar down. People suffering from type II are allowed to eat almost everything but in restriction and in exchange of each other and in limitation. Palatability, variety and aesthetic sense are points that need to be considered while planning their diet. Alternatives should be provided for each restriction. Each meal should be planned for a nutrient dense diet.

People who are suffering from diabetes have more chances of developing other chronic diseases for example hypertension, cardiovascular diseases, stroke, renal diseases, etc. They should be advised to take a diet that is low in fat, salt and cholesterol. They should be provided with a list of food items that they can eat freely. Restrictions on diet make people disheartened and lose hope. They should be encouraged to see the positive side of the picture and the foods in a variety of ways that they are allowed to eat. There are lots of foods that they can enjoy in abundance. They should be advised not to over eat meat items. Exercise can be a lifeline if strict diet restrictions are difficult to follow. Many sweet dishes can be prepared using artificial sweeteners and alternatives. Rice dishes can be used in limitations. Potato can be used in exchange of cereal group. Low fat meat and white meat is better. Oil is better than butter or any kind of saturated fat.

DIET PILLS FOR WEIGHT REDUCTION

Due to increasing incidences of obesity and over-weight through-out the world in general and in the west in particular have led new innovative ideas for weight loss. One such idea is to reduce weight through diet pills which many people find to be easy and convenient to proceed with at home level. Diet pills have actually in different variations remained prevalent since the beginning of previous century. Most of these drugs were either removed or banned for public usage due to their severe or fatal side effects. Currently there is only one anti-obesity Orlistate approved by the FDA and need to be taken through professional guidance. Diet pills either work by suppressing the appetite or affecting fat absorption during digestion. What-ever way they work they are synthetic chemical compounds and therefore cannot be trusted for their total safety especially for long term usage. Improved socio economic conditions and changing lifestyle have all contributed towards rapid increase in chronic obesity and consequently leading to many related chronic diseases e. g. diabetes, hypertension, cardiovascular diseases, etc. It is better to prevent obesity. A person and health care providers and family need to get alert at the onset of overweight leading to obesity. A person who is 15% - 20% over weight for his or her ideal body weight should start looking towards reducing weight in a more health friendly manner rather than proceeding towards obesity and later regretting and taking quick remedial fixes.

Weight loss needed to be achieved in natural ways. Changing one's lifestyle, diet and exercise can contribute positively in achieving this and therefore needed to be taken seriously at this stage. Expecting magical powers through pills can have lifelong impact on overall health and wellbeing of any given individual. Suppressing the appetite may lead towards food nutrient deficiencies to occur. Many claims about the pills to have magical weight reducing powers have not even been tried for authenticity and tested for its total safety. Compromising on one's health and becoming a victim of irresponsible marketing can even cause life-long irreversible damages to the body that could lead to death. Believing in all the tactics of marketing and word of mouth is not going to lead in any kind of right direction. It could only going to ruin one's health. Health is such a great wealth that if once lost cannot be bought with all the might of wealth. One thing is certain that weight loss cannot be achieved through quick fixes and therefore should not be our goal. Approaching the problem and dealing with it in the right way should be our goal which could help us in achieving success in this.

DIET THERAPY FOR POLYCYSTIC KIDNEY DISEASE

Polycystic Kidney Disease or Kidney Failure is mostly a genetic disorder or disease of kidneys and runs in a family. Sometimes polycystic kidney disease is also acquired e. g. due to old age. Poly means many and polycystic kidney disease means, kidneys having many cysts and are filled with fluids making the kidneys to become enlarge. More than twelve million people all around the world are affected by polycystic kidney disease. The Progression of polycystic kidney disease can be slowed down if proper care is taken in the beginning. Initially diet therapy is the only available regiment for people suffering from polycystic kidney disease. A renal failure diet is suggested for patients suffering from polycystic kidney disease, which is low in high biological value protein or foods acquired through animals and is replaced by plant sources of protein to lessen the progression of this disease. Minerals like sodium and potassium are also decreased as they have the capacity to hold more water in the body and patients suffering from advance stages of polycystic kidney disease face difficulty in getting rid of the extra fluid present inside the body. Sources of sodium include common salt and all products that contain common salt, milk and all its products, spinach, etc. Total intake of water and all fluid intake is also restricted according to the stage of polycystic kidney disease. Protein intake, sodium, potassium and fluid intake is restricted according to individual cases of patients suffering from polycystic kidney disease. As the disease advances and progresses the diet therapy need to be followed by dialysis. Dialysis helps in removing all the extra fluid and toxic waste from the bodies of patients suffering from this disease. After initiation of dialysis a patient of polycystic kidney disease is allowed to take increased quantity of high biological value protein as the body is secreting lots of good quality protein through dialysis. Thirdly if the medical team or patients decide to go through available kidney transplant and if everything goes well for the patient as well as the medical team, these patients may fully recover and start taking a regular diet. Lots of researches are being carried out to understand this disease. Better alternatives, cure and treatment methods for people suffering from polycystic kidney disease are being studied to relieve the patients of the sufferings.

JOINT PAIN RELIEF

Arthralgia means joint pain and can be a symptom of injury, infection, allergic reaction or may be a result of many diseases or conditions. Arthritis, gout, lupus, bursitis and many other joint diseases can cause joint pain. Home remedies, over the counter drugs and many available therapies could be used to relieve pain initially. Understanding the underlying causes for this kind of pain may need professional guidance and treatment plans. Joint pain especially knee pain is very common in any given population. Following given examples are few of the tried and tested methods to relieve joint pain.

1.   Over-the-Counter   Drugs   for   example aspirin.

2.   Topical Agents for example chili peppers.

3.   Oil Massage.

4.   Sleeping well and Rest.

5.   Hot Water Bottle.

6.   Exercise and Regular Activity.

7.   Physical Therapy.

8.   Diet Therapy.

9.   Herbal Therapy.

10.   Psychological therapy.

11.   Pain Relieving gels; roll on, ointments, towelettes.

12.   Ice Pack Therapy.

13.   Hypnosis.

14.   Acupuncture.

15.   TENS.

16.   Yoga.

In-depth understanding of most of the above given therapies and recommendations to relieve joint pain at home level can be beneficial if used properly, cautiously and with intervals between each to assess its effects on an individual. Many of the above given list to get relieve from joint pains may need a professional advice and guidance. Each individual may need individualized advice according to him/her stage of the disease as well as practical implications involved with each one.

SIMPLE STEPS TO AVOID CONSTIPATION

If you are feeling constipated and needed relief, many simple home remedies could be used to achieve this. Within a few days' time you could feel normal again. These simple home remedies could be used to achieve this at home level at any given time. Drinking enough water and fluids and eating a diet high in soluble and in-soluble fiber help in keeping the peristaltic movement normal and digestive residue hydrated which helps in keeping constipation at bay. It helps in flushing out the toxins as well as solid wastes from the body. Drinking enough means consuming at least 1500ml 2500ml on a daily basis which is being recommended by health care professionals. Fluid needs depend upon the weather and climate conditions of any given area as well as activity factors, height, weight and age of any given individual. Stop ignoring your body and self and start paying more visits to your bathroom. According to one study 20% of the American population avoids to do this. Ignoring the signs of bowel movement can start showing signs of chronic constipation which could prove to be disastrous in long term. The toxic waste if not relieved when needed could get hardened and dry which could be a cause for great discomfort.

Increasing intake of whole grain cereals, beans, legumes, pulses, lentils, peas, vegetables and fruits can be beneficial for providing protection from chronic constipation as well as improving over-all health.

WISDOM TOOTH

Our teeth are a blessing showered upon us by nature not just for the sake of beauty but for many other factors which help us to stay happy, healthy and lead a normal life. Tooth decay, painful or bleeding gums can prove to be disastrous for our health leading to unhappiness, uneasiness, pain and difficulty in eating and having a negative impact on our overall health and wellbeing. Ignoring the signs of unhealthy teeth could lead to irreversible problems. Whether you are a minor, an adult or a senior citizen, you might have to go through painful scenario and desperately needed help at least once in your lifetime.

Our overall health depends on having healthy teeth. In order to keep our teeth healthy, free from dental carries and cavities, good care, proper nourishment and thorough cleaning is needed. How often to brush our teeth, how to floss our teeth and how to protect and take proper over all care, proper guidance may be needed. Nourishment and diet play a vital role in helping our teeth healthy and well maintained.

Nutrient deficiencies can lead to unhealthy teeth and can lead progressively towards tooth decay, cavities and several abnormal conditions which can impact the overall healthy functioning of teeth. Many foods and many food combinations need to be avoided. e. g. carbonated beverages, too much of sweet and too sticky sweets, synthetic drinks, too much of starchy fruits, vegetables or cereals. Smoking and alcohol drinking are well known causes for tooth decay.

Orthodontics have been striving hard to prevent and correct all kind of irregularities of teeth faced by people of all ages, cultures and socio-economics spectrum. They help them to have braces if needed, where needed and whenever needed. People with crooked teeth can avail their expertise to overcome their existing problems. These experts will be able to diagnose the problem and make proper plan for its treatment based on individual needs and desires. These specialists also help in correcting the jaw line and helps in straitening person's teeth by the use of braces, retainers, etc.

Then we also have Prosthodontics who help people who are suffering from various dental problems and providing them with proper treatment needed. People, who have been suffering from any kind of oral malfunction, discomfort, missing teeth, etc., can look towards them for advice and treatment. They can look forward to improving their existing condition by visiting a dentist who will be able to provide them with timely medical care needed. They also provide with aesthetic restoration as well as replacements needed. In other words they help in beautifying the smiles and improving the looks. This is a known fact that many people visit dentist not for any kind of treatment for diseases but for cosmetic purposes. To look beautiful, feel beautiful and smile beautiful.

Family Dentist can be a great help for the whole families. No need to have each dentist for each individual of the family. Families can have family dentist who can look after all the needs and requirements of the families. Families need to look for family dentist close to their living areas who could fulfill the requirements of all. Keeping the teeth happy and healthy is better than regretting and suffering. People need to take wisdom tooth from these dentists to keep themselves and their families aware of all needed to be known so that they do not have to face all the difficulties later on. Your dentist is the best to provide you with this. If you have not asked him yet please do ask him now so that you may live in peace later on.

10. *FRUITS FOR GOOD HEALTH*

Fruits have proven record of providing innumerable health, healing and beauty benefits. They can be found in all shapes, sizes, colors, aroma, texture, shades and varieties. They are best if used as a snack or as a substitute for a skipped meal. They are loaded with minerals, vitamins, natural sugars, complex carbohydrates, and soluble and in-soluble fiber. They are much easier to incorporate into many creative healthy recipes but it is always better to eat these in the raw form and therefore their salads could be prepared and best used at meal times. A long list of these have been searched and listed here to add variety in taste and texture of each meal. Fruits are considered food of the heavens and we should be thankful for their presence in the worldly abode. We must try to consume as much fruits in our lifetime as possible as these are mostly free of all the artificial colors, flavors and chemical compounds and are available in the most natural forms.

1.   APPLE

2.   BANANA

3.   ORANGE

4.   MANGO

5.   POMEGRANATE

6.   PLUM

7.   PEACH

8.   KIWI

9.   LIME

10.   PINEAPPLE

11.   STRAW BERRY

12.   GUAVA

13.   BLUE BERRIES

14.   BLACK BERRIES

15.   FIGS

16.   CANTALOUPE

17.   WATER MELON

18.   CHEEKO

19.   CHERRIES

20.   TANGERINE

21.   GRAPES

22. LEECHEE

23. DATES

24. PEAR

25. APPRICOTS

26. AVOCADO

27. PAPAYA

28. LEMON

29. RASP BERRY

30. GRAPE FRUIT

31. NECTARINES

32. CURRANTS

33. GOOSE BERRY

34. HONEYDEW MELON

35. RUBARBS

36. CRAN BERRY

37. ACAI BERRY

38. CHERIMOYA

39. LOQUAT

40. KUMQUAT

41. CHOKE BERRY

42. JACK FRUIT

43. PASSION FRUIT

44. RUM RUNNER

45. CARIBBEAN

46. MARGARITA

47. WILD BERRY

48. TOMATO

49. BREAD FRUIT

50. PERSIMMON

51. POMELO

52. SALAL BERRY

53. SATSUMA

54. STAR FRUIT

55. UGLI FRUIT

56. ROCK MELON

57. CANARY MELON

58. MANDARIN

59. LEGUME

60. JUJUBE

61. JAMBUL

62. JETTA MELON

63. HUCKLE BERRY

64. BIL BERRY

65. CHERIMOYA

66. CLEMENTINE

67. CLOUD BERRY

68. DAMSON

69. DRAGON FRUIT

70. DURIAN

71. ELDER BERRY

72. FEIJOA

73. MUSK MELON

74. RED MOMBIN

75. KUNDONG

76. PULASAN

77. RIBERRY

78. STRAW BERRY GUAVA

79. MELON PEAR

80. SONCOYA

81. ABIU

82. LANGSAT

83. SAFOU

84. MORINDA

85. GOJI BERRIES

86. DRAGON BERRIES

87. SOURSOP

88. MANGOSTEEN RAISINS

89. PLANTAIN

90. CLEMENTINES

91. MULBERRIES

92. PRUNES

93. BLACK CURRANTS

94. RAMBUTAN

95. AFRICAN CUCUMBER

96. QUINCES

97. CRABAPPLES

98. CHOKE BERRIES

99. ARBUTUS UNEDO

100. ROSE APPLE

101. CUSTARD APPLE

102. PLUM MANGO

103. LANGSART

104. LOGAN

105. SANTOL

106. TAMARIND

107. TANGELOS

108. OLIVES

www.ingramcontent.com/pod-product-compliance
Lightning Source LLC
Chambersburg PA
CBHW060332290526
45793CB00003B/602